HOMEOPATHIC PRESCRIBING

Keats books on homeopathic subjects

Who Is Your Doctor and Why?
by Alonzo J. Shadman, M.D.

The Bach Flower Remedies (Three Books in One Volume)
by Edward Bach, M.D. & F. J. Wheeler, M.D.

The Healing Art of Homeopathy
by Edward C. Hamlyn, M.D.

The Medical Discoveries of Edward Bach, Physician
by Nora Weeks

Handbook of the Bach Flower Remedies
by Philip M. Chancellor

Materia Medica of New Homeopathic Remedies
by O. A. Julian, M.D.

Homeopathic Prescribing
by Noel J. Pratt, M.D.

Homeopathy in Practice
by Douglas Borland, M.D.

Introduction to Homeopathic Medicine
by Hamish Boyd, M.D.

A Guide to Medicinal Plants
by Paul Schauenberg & Ferdinand Paris

Homeopathic Prescribing

NOEL J. PRATT, M.D.
MRCS, LRCP, MFHom

With an Appendix on the Constitutional Remedies by
MARION GRAY, M.D., BM, BCh, MRCGP, MFHom

Keats Publishing, Inc. New Canaan, Connecticut

Note: The spelling of homeopathy herein follows the British style as it appears in the original text. Where new material has been added (cover text, bibliography, introductory copy, list of companies making and selling homeopathic products, etc.), Americanized spelling has been used.

Homeopathic Prescribing

Published by arrangement with Beaconsfield Publishers, Ltd., Beaconsfield, Bucks, U.K.

ISBN: 0-87983-325-4 (previously ISBN 0-906584-03-5)
Library of Congress Catalog Card Number 82-084364

Printed in the United States of America

Keats Publishing, Inc.
27 Pine Street, New Canaan, Connecticut

Dedicated to the memory of
Francis Hervey Bodman,
MD, ChB, MRCS, LRCP, FRCPsych, DPM, FFHom
in gratitude for his many writings.

INTRODUCTION

This book is intended for the student of homoeopathy who requires short lists of remedies for most of the common ailments.

In composing these lists I have referred to the works of other authors, in addition to drawing on my own experience of homoeopathic prescribing in thirty years in the National Health Service. I gratefully acknowledge my main sources of reference:

Dr C. M. Boger's *Synoptic Key of the Materia Medica*, Dr J. H. Clarke's *The Prescriber*, Dr D. M. Gibson's *Homoeopathic First Aid*, Dr R. Hughes' *Principles and Practice of Homoeopathy*, Dr J. T. Kent's *Repertory*, Drs Neatby and Stonham's *Manual of Homoeopathic Therapeutics* and Dr Margaret Tyler's *Drug Pictures*.

It is assumed that the reader has some basic knowledge of homoeopathy and will not need instruction on potency and dosage. Other readers who wish to have more information may like to read Dr Clarke's fifty page introduction to the last edition of his book, *The Prescriber*; it is one of the best explanations of the subject.

This book is primarily for qualified physicians, who will know when investigation and other treatment is needed. The book can, of course, be bought by others who are not medically qualified but require the information for the benefit of themselves, their families and friends. To such persons I say: homoeopathy is of great value as first aid and for minor diseases, but if there is any doubt of the significance of the symptoms and signs of the disease for which a remedy is sought, be sure to obtain the opinion of a qualified physician. You may find the homoeopathic remedy a valuable supplement to other treatment.

The list of symptoms, signs and diagnoses is presented in alphabetical order. The sections are confined to one page for ease of reference and to avoid any confusion which might arise from long lists of remedies, including some which are seldom used. In each section the remedies are presented in alphabetical order; this is better than trying to arrange them in order of importance, about which opinions would differ. Lay terms are not always included – sometimes they are deliberately omitted. For example, 'Spots' would be an unsatisfactory section; the prescriber must know what variety of spots is in question. Relatively vague terms such as Sore Throat have no separate sections, because the reader will need to make a more precise diagnosis, such as Tonsillitis, Pharyngitis, Laryngitis, or Tracheitis, and then refer to the appropriate page.

I have carefully considered the suggestion that the subject matter should be presented under the headings of the anatomical systems most involved in each disease. I have decided not to do so, because the book does not pretend to be a systematic textbook in that sense, but essentially a handbook for quick refreshing of the memory.

The brief notes after each remedy will not always be sufficient to select the right one without further thought; these few symptoms and signs are in the nature of reminders, to encourage further thought. It is usually necessary to take into account not only the main symptoms and signs, but also the physical and temperamental characteristics of the patient, and the various factors which make the disease better or worse.

Critics may object that the presentation of short lists of remedies will encourage prescribers to dodge the work of formal repertorisation on paper in the Kentian manner. There are times when full repertorisation is necessary, but there are other times when personal experience enables a simpler way of selecting the similimum, especially when aided by a handbook such as this.

It will be noticed that there are only a few sections concerning mental symptoms and the various moods and temperaments. The main reason is that to include them all would make the book unwieldy. In Kent's *Repertory*, for example, there are eighty-four major rubrics in the ninety-four pages devoted to 'Mind'. Therefore no attempt has been made to mention all of them.

I refrain from recommending any particular potencies, and merely state that, in my experience, the low potencies are most useful in acute disease, taken fairly frequently until relief is obtained, and the high potencies are most useful in chronic disease, taken once or twice a day until improvement is noticed. When the general health is affected, I find a constitutional remedy is indicated.

Patients sometimes need a 'local' or 'organ' remedy to begin treatment, followed by the constitutional remedy to complete treatment and to restore good health; at other times it is advisable to begin treatment with a single dose of the constitutional remedy and follow immediately with a course of the 'local' remedy.

Strange, rare and peculiar symptoms are mentioned, just as in the clinical situation patients sometimes describe their troubles in strange, rare and peculiar terms. In teaching hospitals these are usually ignored because they do not fit into the textbook descriptions of disease. Many doctors hardly hear them because they seem to be irrelevant to prescribing, but when they are used for selecting the homoeopathic remedy, their value is great.

The list of subjects is deliberately not comprehensive; most of the infectious, contagious and notifiable diseases have been omitted, because if they are not treated (and when necessary notified) on conventional lines, allegations of negligence are possible. Nevertheless, homoeopathic remedies can be valuable additional treatment, especially in convalescence and for any sequelae. Readers will probably consider there is room for improvement in the book, and that some additions and corrections will be needed. I shall be grateful for any comments which can be acted on if the demand for the book is sufficient to justify a second edition.

Homoeopathy cannot, in my opinion, reverse degenerative diseases, but experience of its use does seem to justify the hope that it may restrain degenerative processes or even halt them, by improving the general health.

Dr Marion Gray's list of constitutional remedies and the main indications for them is a welcome Appendix to the book. Whenever no 'local' or 'organ' remedy is clearly indicated, reference to the list of constitutional remedies will usually enable the choice to be made with confidence.

I am grateful for the many helpful comments by my friends, Dr Hamish Boyd, Dr Marianne Harling, Dr Alastair Jack, Dr Marion Gray and Mr John Ainsworth, MPS, who read the first drafts for the book.

Homoeopathic knowledge continues to grow, as is shown by the recent publication of the *Materia Medica of New Homoeopathic Remedies* by Dr O. A. Julian of Paris, in which there are seventy-eight new remedies described and recent additional information about twenty-eight other remedies.

Every physician should strive to record all that he or she learns from experience, as well as from conversations and from reading. The interleaved pages of this book are suitable for recording such knowledge.

N.J.P.

CONTENTS

ACNE

In addition to the usual advice on diet, skin care and general hygiene, these remedies should be considered:

Belladonna for acne in full-blooded, red-faced persons.

Hepar Sul. when pustules are a prominent feature.

Pulsatilla for acne in pale blondes of either sex.

Silica when there is much scarring.

Staphylococcin if the response to other remedies is slow.

Sulphur for long-standing obstinate cases.

ACNE ROSACEA

Arsenicum Album when there is noticeable desquamation and burning sensations.

Belladonna for full-blooded, red-faced persons.

Lachesis when caused by oral contraceptives; in addition to the eruption, there is burning of the face, worse in hot rooms and worse after taking alcohol.

Nux Vomica when there is an above-average intake of alcohol, especially of spirits.

Rhus Tox. when the nose is red, shiny and swollen, and there is a tendency to develop pustules.

Sulphur Iod. when the face is dry and red, and develops pustules.

ADENOIDS, ENLARGED

Bacillinum when there is a family tendency to enlarged adenoids, and especially if there is a family history of tuberculosis.

Barium Carb. for children who are under-developed physically and also mentally backward.

Calc. Carb. for pale, fat children with cold, clammy feet, and sweating of the head at night.

Calc. Phos. for thin children with large troublesome adenoids.

Psorinum with itchy skin and offensive sweat.

Sulphur for the child who is always hungry, especially about eleven in the morning, and has a marked dislike of hot baths; for adenoids (and tonsils) which are so large as to cause some degree of obstruction.

AGGRESSION

Belladonna for sudden and violent aggression, with an 'inclination' to bite.

Nux Vomica when the patient is easily offended, reacts irritably, and develops tension headaches and dyspepsia.

Sepia for the occasional episodes of aggression in contrast to the usual depression and apathy.

Staphisagria when aggressive tendencies arise from resentment or anger which is more or less repressed, with consequent physical repercussions.

Sulphur for persons with aggressive tendencies concerning institutions rather than people – social reformers with strange, even grandiose, ideas: 'burning with zeal, and itching for action'.

ALCOHOLISM

Some form of psychotherapy is always needed, as well as advice on diet and habits.

Aconite for episodes of fear and delirium.

Antim. Tart. for nausea and vomiting, especially if there is also bronchial catarrh.

Arsenicum Album for restlessness and mental aberrations.

Capsicum when the main symptom is gastritis.

Cinchona wants to be alone for solitary drinking.

Crotalus Horridus when vomiting of blood occurs. (That may necessitate admission to hospital.)

Lachesis for the voluble social over-drinker.

Nux Vomica for hangovers and morning vomiting, especially after brandy.

Quercus to help to suppress the craving.

Sulphur will drink almost anything, indiscriminately.

Tuberculinum when drinking leads to violence.

Zinc Met. with twitching and trembling.

ANGER, AND AILMENTS AFTER ANGER

Aconite for anger originating in fright – for example, the situation after a road accident.

Chamomilla for anger in the young, and in the old – the remedy for cantankerous behaviour in 'second childhood'.

Colocynth for anger leading to colic and neuralgia.

Crocus for anger with violence, with quick repentance.

Hepar Sul. easily roused to vehemence and rapid speech.

Ignatia unreasonable anger leading to a variety of hysterical manifestations.

Nux Vomica irritability and anger, causing dyspepsia and other troubles.

Staphisagria suppressed anger and indignation, leading to headaches and other pains.

NOTES

NOTES

ANGINA PECTORIS

Aconite when the pain causes much alarm, and especially if there is also tingling in the arm or hand.

Cactus with the classical sensation of an iron band round the chest, 'as in a vice'.

Carbo Veg. for pseudo-angina, caused by excess wind in the stomach, or by too big a meal.

Glonoine with much throbbing.

Lachesis with a sense of constriction in the neck as well as in the chest.

Latrodectus with rapid pulse, nausea and vomiting.

Lilium Tig. when the heart feels squeezed, alternately grasped and relaxed.

Spigelia with marked palpitations, noticeable to observers.

ANUS, FISSURE OF

Aesculus with burning soreness and pain in the back.

Chamomilla with haemorrhoids.

Graphites with painful smarting and soreness.

Nitric Acid with sharp cutting pains and prickings.

Ratanhia with burning after defaecation, and sharp stabs as if with a knife.

Silica when healing is slow.

Thuja with various other anal and rectal symptoms and pain causing frequency of micturition.

Tuberculinum with a sense of pressure in the rectum and leading to diarrhoea.

ANUS, ITCHING OF (PRURITIS ANI)

Alumina with prickling as if by pins.

Ambra Grisea with itching of the pudenda.

Antim. Crud. with smarting, worse at night.

Ignatia with violent itching and crawling sensations, but not due to threadworms.

Nitric Acid worse when walking in the open air, and after stool.

Petroleum worse when riding in cars, and worse at night in bed.

Sulphur with prolapse of the anus as well as the itching.

APPETITE, CRAVINGS

Argentum Nit. for sweet things and salty things.

Calc. Carb. for salt.

Carbo Anim. for sour and refreshing items of diet.

China for something, but does not know what.

Hepar Sul. for sour or highly flavoured pungent things such as curry.

Ignatia for indigestible things, especially in pregnancy.

Natrum Mur. for salt.

Nux Vomica for brandy.

Phosphorus for sugar, but not for fats.

Psorinum appetite much increased for anything.

Pulsatilla for beer.

Sepia for vinegar.

Silica for cold uncooked foods.

Sulphur for fats and for sugar.

APPETITE, LOSS OF

Calc. Carb. especially does not want meat.

Ignatia loss of appetite for everything.

Nux Vomica appetite spoilt by bitter taste in the mouth, and a tongue with a thick yellow coating.

Lycopodium fullness after a few mouthfuls, as if too much has already been eaten.

Pulsatilla little appetite, and no thirst.

Rhus Tox. loss of appetite for everything.

APPREHENSION

Argentum Nit. apprehension leading to diarrhoea.

Arsenicum Album with restlessness – paces up and down.

Carbo Veg. especially on waking – and wants fresh air.

Gelsemium unable to act – 'paralysed' by apprehension.

Lycopodium dreads tasks like making speeches, but when the time comes, rises to the occasion.

Medorrhinum with the feeling that time goes too slowly.

Phosphoric Acid a mixture of apprehension and indifference.

Plumbum with impaired memory, and fear of forgetting words.

Silica with undue sensitivity to music.

Thuja with headache like a nail being driven into the head.

NOTES

NOTES

ARTHRITIS, ACUTE

Apis with much swelling of the soft tissues, and redness, like a bee sting.

Arnica especially helpful when arthritic joints are bruised by blows and falls.

Bryonia for acute exacerbations, when no relief is obtained from movement – in contrast to Rhus Tox.

Dulcamara when noticeably worse after cold and damp, as from unaired beds, as well as from damp weather.

Ledum after injections – when corticosteroid injections have not been as helpful as expected.

Pulsatilla pains go from joint to joint, and are variable and unpredictable.

ARTHRITIS, CHRONIC

Argentum Nit. for the anxious person who tends to move too fast and has accidents which aggravate the arthritis.

Aurum Met. in homoeopathic potency, as valuable as the conventional injections, and without risk of dermatitis.

Calc. Fluor. when exostoses develop in association with arthritis.

Calc. Phos. when arthritis is initiated or made worse during pregnancy.

Causticum especially when contractures develop or threaten.

Colchicum for gouty arthritis.

Kali Bich. for joint pains alternating with catarrhal or gastric symptoms.

Nux Vomica for associated muscle spasms as distinct from muscle stiffness.

Rhus Tox. when there is muscle stiffness protecting the affected joints – better after moving about a little.

Ruta when ganglia are present.

Sepia for menopausal arthritis.

Sulphur for psoriatic arthritis.

ASTHMA

It is impossible to condense the many remedies for asthma on to one page, but a short list may be helpful. In addition to the constitutional remedies and the nosodes the following should be considered:

Antim. Tart. with wheezing so loud that it can be heard in the next room.

Arsenicum Album with restlessness.

Ipecacuanha with catarrh of the nose and throat, and with scanty sputum.

Kali Carb. especially if attacks begin between 3 a.m. and 5 a.m.

Lobelia with nausea and a tendency to heart failure.

Natrum Sul. when there is a tendency to salt and water retention and morning diarrhoea, and the asthma is worse in damp weather.

Veratrum Viride when a condition similar to shock develops – cold sweat, nausea and vomiting.

BACKACHE

These are a few of the many remedies which are valuable for back pain and also for associated weakness of the back.

Arnica for bruises and for sensations similar to bruises.

Arsenicum Album backache with restlessness – cannot find a comfortable position.

Calc. Carb. worse while sitting.

Kali Carb. for backache and weakness persisting after pregnancy and labour.

Nux Vomica with tension in the back muscles, limiting flexion of the spine.

Phosphoric Acid when weakness is more complained of than pain.

Rhus Tox. if stiffness is marked, especially on first movements, and better after continued movement.

NOTES

NOTES

BELCHING

Argentum Nit. loud copious and painless belching.

Carbo An. with a sense of pressure, and with choking.

Carbo Veg. with distension of the stomach.

Carbolic Acid with nervous dyspepsia.

Mag. Carb. with vomiting of sour fluid.

Mag. Phos. small belches without relief of discomfort.

Mancinella with burning sensations rising from the stomach to the throat.

Phosphorus desires cold drinks.

Pulsatilla belching with a taste of the food of the last meal.

Sulphur belching with particles of food and with an unpleasant smell.

BLEPHARITIS

Apis for acute cases with much redness, burning, stinging, and swelling of the eyelids.

Belladonna also for the acute stage, especially if the eyes are dry and hot, and the pupils are dilated.

Hepar Sul. when the eyelids are stuck together after sleep, and when the pain threshold is low.

Merc. Sol. when there is much exudate, and when blepharospasm is pronounced.

BLISTERS AND VESICLES

Arsenicum Album burning sensations, better for warmth.

Cantharis for burns and scalds to prevent the development of blisters.

Causticum for vesicles, fissures and warts – with a raw feeling, as if the skin were grazed.

Lachesis vesicles with a purple or blue tinge, leaving ulcers, especially on the left.

Mezereum especially when the scalp is involved and when thick scabs are formed.

Natrum Mur. for blisters or vesicles on the lips.

Nitric Acid with pricking sensations.

Phosphorus with burning sensations and fidgeting.

Ranunculus for shingles on the chest wall.

Rhus Tox. when urticaria is severe and the lesions almost look like blisters.

BOILS AND FURUNCLES

Diabetes and other causes should be detected or excluded in case other treatment is essential. Then the following remedies may be considered:

Apis with much redness and swelling around the boil.

Arnica for boils in sensitive parts, with bruised sensation.

Arsenicum Album with burning sensations.

Belladonna when boils are surrounded by bright red 'angry' areas.

Graphites with dry skin, and insufficient sweat to keep it healthy.

Hepar Sul. when every little skin injury turns septic and when blisters develop into boils.

Lachesis unusually painful boils with a bluish tinge.

Merc. Sol. for furuncles in the ears.

Phytolacca for boils on the back.

Pyrogen for angry spreading boils.

Silica for boils which develop slowly and heal slowly, especially in chilly persons.

Staphylococcin for furunculosis.

Sulphur when a series of boils occurs, especially if the patient scratches a lot.

Tarentula purplish boils with severe burning and stinging.

BONE PAINS

Aurum Met. burning and boring pains in bones, with redness and swelling – if it has been proved *not* to be due to osteomyelitis.

Eupatorium bone pains during influenza.

Hekla Lava painful lumps on bones – exostoses.

Kali Bich. for pains in small spots, especially in or on the bones of the head.

Mezereum rheumatic pains in bones, worse at night.

Phosphorus burning pains in bones, especially of the mandible – similar to the 'phossy jaw' of phosphorus poisoning.

Rhododendron worse before stormy weather – for persons who can thus foretell rain and thunder.

Ruta pains associated with sprains.

Silica for children who are thin and weak and complain of bone pains.

NOTES

NOTES

BREAST, PAIN IN

Asterias Rubens for drawing pains associated with cancer – as supplementary treatment.

Belladonna with throbbing.

Bellis Perennis also for pain of breast cancer.

Bryonia with heaviness, better for gentle pressure and support.

Calc. Carb. pain before periods.

Conium pain before periods, with lumpiness.

Graphites for painful cracked nipples, in addition to local treatment.

Hepar Sul. when slight injuries lead to suppuration or inflammation.

Lachesis pains worse on waking.

Merc. Sol. pains worse at night.

Phytolacca for mastitis, with the characteristic swelling and lumpiness.

Pulsatilla for pains which come and go unpredictably, causing tears.

Silica undue pain while nursing the baby.

BRONCHITIS

Aconite in the early stages.

Ammon. Carb. in the later stages, when it is difficult to raise the sputum.

Antim. Tart. when there is loud rattling in the chest.

Arsenicum Album worse at night – with much coughing but little sputum.

Belladonna in the early stages, with hot dry skin and red face.

Bryonia dry hacking cough with pain in the chest.

Carbo Veg. for older persons with a tendency to cyanosis.

Causticum with stress incontinence of urine.

Conium short dry cough with tickling behind the sternum.

Hepar Sul. with profuse yellow sputum.

Hyoscyamus the cough begins as soon as the patient lies down.

Ipecacuanha cough leading to nausea and gagging.

Kali Bich. when the sputum is tenacious and stringy.

Merc. Sol. with a tendency to extra sweating.

Pulsatilla worse lying down and in a warm room.

Rumex with soreness in the trachea and behind the sternum; worse in cold air.

Senega for painful rattling in the chest – sputum hard to raise.

Stannum bronchitis with a weak feeling in the chest.

Sulphur for the later stages of bronchitis, when the cough is worse in bed at night.

BRUISES

Arnica the remedy most often used for bruises, especially when muscles are involved.

Bellis for bruises of the breast.

Hamamelis when the skin over a bruise is broken, also for bruises of varicose veins.

Hypericum for bruises of parts especially rich in nerve endings – the fingers and toes.

Ruta for injuries involving bruises of bones and of tendons.

BUNIONS

Antim. Crud. for elderly persons with tender feet, worse in warm rooms.

Benzoic Acid especially for persons with gout as well as bunions.

Kali Iod. when there is also a tendency to chilblains.

Rhododendron when bunions are more painful before storms.

Silica when the bunions are hard and not much inflamed.

BURNS AND SCALDS

Cantharis usually the best first aid, in the form of lotion.

Causticum for painful burn scars.

Hamamelis can also be used as a lotion as first aid.

Hepar Sul. for burns which have become infected.

Kali Bich. for second degree burns – the equivalent of ulcers.

Urtica for persistent stinging sensations.

NOTES

NOTES

CATARRH, CHRONIC NASAL

Obstinate cases often require constitutional remedies as **Pulsatilla, Sulphur, Psorinum, Tuberculinum, Carcinosinum** and **Morgan Co**. These remedies are usually chosen on the personal history, but at other times the family history is of value in deciding which is needed.

Arsenicum Iod. in weakly debilitated persons with drippy nose and sore nostrils.

Aurum Met. with soreness of the nasal bones, and much depression.

Graphites when there is also constipation, and skin eruptions around the nostrils.

Hydrastis for constant post-nasal drip and eustachian catarrh.

Kali Bich. with yellow or white stringy catarrh.

Natrum Mur. fluent catarrh, intermittent, variable in quantity from day to day; much sneezing.

Sanguinaria with stinging and tickling in the nose, and some swelling, inside and outside.

CHICKEN POX

In addition to the usual nursing care, the following remedies should be considered:

Antim. Crud. the patient cries if washed or touched, or even if looked at.

Antim. Tart. wants much attention and is very irritable.

Pulsatilla weeps easily; has little thirst.

Rhus Tox. with itching and restlessness; to encourage the drying of the vesicles.

Sulphur hot, eats little but drinks lots.

One can also consider treatment in a sequential scheme:

Aconite in the initial stages.

Rhus Tox. when the blisters form.

Merc. Sol. during convalescence.

Varicellinum when sequelae persist.

CHILBLAINS

Agaricus more painful when cold.

Apis with stinging sensations, even when they are not in contact with anything.

Arsenicum Album with burning sensations.

Calc. Carb. in pale and obese persons, better when cold.

Graphites for broken chilblains, with a gluey exudate.

Kali Iod. when there is much swelling around the chilblains.

Nux Vomica for persons in sedentary occupations, underweight, and dislike of windy weather.

Petroleum when the skin has broken – and when the finger tips are cracked.

Pulsatilla more painful in warm rooms and in bed, and particularly after exposure to radiant heat.

Rhus Tox. when there is blistering associated with chilblains.

Tamus when the desire to scratch is irresistible.

Zincum Met. for chilblains which are worse after rubbing, especially in persons with fidgety feet.

COCCYDYNIA (PAIN IN COCCYX)

Antim. Tart. with a sensation of a heavy load on the coccyx, dragging the body down.

Apis burning and stinging pain.

Causticum drawing or bruised sensation.

Cicuta tearing and jerking pain.

Hypericum after a fall.

Kali Bich. pain worse when sitting and when touched.

Silica with constipation.

Zincum Met. with fidgety feet.

NOTES

NOTES

COLIC, INTESTINAL

Belladonna with distension of the transverse colon, with relief when 'doubled up'.

Bryonia better when lying still, and worse from heat.

Chamomilla worse at night, especially during teething.

Cina flatulent colic in older children, with or without infestation by worms.

Cocculus flatulent colic during menstruation.

Colocynth sharp 'cutting' colic, better for bending double, can't keep still – writhes and twists.

Dioscerea colic worse for pressure, better for straightening the spine and for walking about.

Mag. Phos. with sharp cramping pains, better for heat.

Plumbum with obstinate constipation and other symptoms similar to lead poisoning.

Stannum when the pain comes on slowly and passes slowly.

Staphisagria colic due to suppressed anger or indignation.

Veratrum Album severe colic leading to symptoms of shock.

COLITIS

These remedies are worth considering for colitis, whether it be mucous colitis, ulcerative colitis or irritable colon.

Argentum Nit. worse when anticipating any kind of ordeal.

Arsenicum Album worse after midnight.

Cantharis with urinary symptoms as well.

Colchicum watery stools.

Colocynth with much colic.

Graphites for obese patients, with offensive flatus.

Kali Sul. worse in the evenings.

Merc. Corr. with blood as well as mucus.

Merc. Sol. with much mucus.

Natrum Sul. worse in the mornings.

Sulphur worse early in the mornings – about 5 a.m.

Veratrum Album copious stools causing faintness.

COMMON COLD

Aconite in the early stage – in the first night.

Allium Cepa with much sneezing and watering of the eyes.

Arsenicum Album with watery catarrh causing sore nostrils.

Euphrasia with irritating tears but bland nasal catarrh.

Ferrum Phos. with nose bleeding.

Gelsemium when the onset is rapid, with chills running up and down the spine.

Hepar Sul. in later stages when the catarrh is thick and yellow.

Kali Iod. if the patient is hot and cold alternately, with a red nose and pain in the forehead.

Mag. Mur. with marked loss of taste and smell.

Mercurius with much sweating, salivation and thick catarrh.

Natrum Mur. when there is much sneezing in the morning.

Nux Vomica fluent nasal catarrh in the day and little at night, and much irritability and intolerance.

Pulsatilla intermittent catarrh, no thirst and better out of doors.

Sanguinaria watery catarrh and a tickling dry cough.

Silica slow onset, slow recovery and with sinusitis.

COMPLEXION

Sometimes a patient's facial appearance is a valuable clue to the choice of a remedy – provided that the symptoms and signs confirm that choice.

Alumina an unhealthy 'earthy' appearance.

Apis when the face is swollen and red.

Arsenicum Album bluish rings around the eyes.

Belladonna bright red.

Calc. Carb. pale and wrinkled.

Gelsemium flushed and congested, with heavy upper eyelids.

Lachesis distended veins and a cyanotic tinge.

Lycopodium wrinkled forehead and pale face.

Phosphorus a 'fresh' red complexion.

Platinum sallow or 'earthy'.

Sepia sallow, brown and with darkened eyelids.

Sulphur red-faced.

Thuja warts and other lumpy lesions.

Veratrum Album the 'Hippocratic' facial appearance of shock and collapse.

NOTES

NOTES

CONCUSSION

Homoeopathic remedies are valuable as first aid after concussion, and are also valuable for the sequelae.

Arnica especially when there is visible bruising.

Cicuta when there are any convulsions or muscle twitchings.

Helleborus when headache persists and is 'stupefying'.

Hypericum if the head is extremely sensitive.

Kali Phos. with insomnia persisting.

Natrum Mur. when depression persists.

CONJUNCTIVITIS

If there is any doubt concerning the cause of conjunctivitis, the opinion of an ophthalmologist should be obtained. In simple cases, in addition to local treatment, homoeopathic remedies can help.

Aconite in the early stages, with injection of the conjunctival blood vessels.

Alumina with dryness.

Apis in acute cases, with chemosis.

Argentum Nit. with muco-purulent discharge.

Arsenicum Album with burning tears – almost a corrosive feeling.

Belladonna with dilation of the pupils.

Euphrasia much watering, with burning and with involvement of the edges of the eyelids.

Pulsatilla conjunctivitis associated with weeping, and much rubbing of the eyes causing inflammation.

Rhus Tox. for involvement of the eyes in cases of shingles.

Silica for the conjunctivitis persisting after injury by foreign bodies.

Sulphur redness of the conjunctivae, not necessarily infected; with hot sensations, worse at night.

CONSTIPATION

In addition to advice on diet and exercise and encouraging a good bowel habit, homoeopathic remedies can be helpful.

Aesculus when there is a sensation of fullness in the rectum even after a motion.

Alumen when the stools are very hard and cause bleeding.

Alumina when there is no urging, but eventually a soft stool with incomplete emptying of the rectum.

Bryonia when the stools are large, hard and dry, in spite of drinking large quantities of fluids.

Calc. Carb. when the patient paradoxically feels better when constipated.

Lycopodium when there are rumblings in the bowels, but no action.

Nitric Acid with painful defaecation resulting in bleeding, and with the sensation of sharp sticks in the rectum.

Nux Vomica for sedentary workers with ineffectual urging; even after a motion the rectum never feels empty.

Opium for 'lazy' bowels with little peristalsis.

Silica when the stool is low in the rectum but hard to pass.

CONVULSIONS

There is little one can do at the time of a convulsion apart from maintaining the airway and preventing injury, but homoeopathic remedies can be helpful in reducing the recurrence of and the severity of the convulsions.

Aconite when caused by fright, and during fevers.

Aethusa with gastroenteritis, especially if there is intolerance of cow's milk.

Belladonna convulsions during fever, with very flushed face, staring eyes and dilated pupils.

Chamomilla during teething, especially if accompanied by anger.

Cicuta with twitchings, jerkings and vertigo.

Cuprum Met. for convulsions caused by the paroxysms of whooping cough, and with cramps and spasms of fingers.

Glonoine after too much exposure to the sun.

Ignatia after punishment and other emotional upsets.

Nux Vomica convulsions preceded by irritability, and sometimes caused by indigestion.

Zinc Sul. in infants with pale face and sunken fontanelle.

NOTES

NOTES

COUGH

Such a common symptom; but a lot of careful thought is required before it can be treated accurately. If persistent, investigations may be needed to establish a precise diagnosis. The following list of remedies is only a sample of the many which are needed from time to time.

Ammon. Carb. productive cough, waking the patient in the night.

Antim. Tart. much rattling in the chest.

Bryonia with pain in the chest as in pleurisy.

Calc. Carb. with tickling provoking the cough.

Causticum dryness, rawness and hoarseness.

Coccus Cacti with a sensitive throat and paroxysmal cough.

Drosera paroxysmal cough with laryngitis or laryngeal spasm.

Ipecacuanha choking cough leading to gagging, nausea and vomiting.

Kali Bich. with stringy sputum.

Kali Carb. with lumpy sputum.

Phosphorus dry racking cough, worse when talking.

Pulsatilla worse in a warm room, better in the open air.

Rumex worse on changing from warm air to cold.

Senega viscid sputum.

Sepia productive cough at night, but little in the day.

Spongia paroxysmal dry cough sounding like a bark.

Sticta dry night cough.

CRAMP

Arnica for cramps which occur when fatigued.

Calc. Carb. for patients who are overweight, pale and 'flabby'.

Camphor for cramps in the calves, with icy coldness of the feet.

Colchicum for cramps in the soles.

Cuprum Met. for cramps beginning as twitches.

Nux Vomica for cramps occurring at night.

Mag. Phos. for writer's cramp in the fingers.

Veratrum Album for cramps occurring as a result of diarrhoea and vomiting – similar to cholera.

CROUP

Croup was the popular name for diphtheria, which has now almost been eradicated. But croupy coughs occur quite often, and these remedies should be considered:

Aconite in the early stages of fevers, especially if brought on by exposure to cold air.

Agaricus for nervy twitchy children – similar to chorea.

Antim. Tart. with rattling sounds in the chest as well.

Belladonna with fever, red face, dry skin and mouth.

Hepar Sul. when croup develops after midnight.

Ignatia when the croup has been brought on by fright or other emotion.

Iodum with wheezing 'sawing' respiration; the child tends to grasp the throat.

Kali Bich. with tough stringy phlegm.

Lachesis waking the patient from sleep.

Sambucus rough sibilant wheezing – and more sweat in the day than when asleep.

Spongia with a hoarse dry barking cough.

CYSTITIS

True cystitis is due to infection, and antibiotic or chemotherapeutic treatment is usually advisable. When infection is resistant, the homoeopathic nosode of the infecting organism can be expected to cure. At other times, so-called cystitis is an irritation of the bladder and urethra; for example, oxaluria after eating too many strawberries. Advice on hygiene may also be appropriate.

Apis frequent micturition with sharp stinging pains.

Belladonna during fever, with concentrated urine.

Benzoic Acid when the urine smells like a dirty stable.

Berberis with turbid urine and a slimy mucous sediment.

Cantharis frequency, and much burning pain.

Causticum frequency, and dribbling leaking at other times.

Dulcamara for cystitis due to chilling in cold damp weather.

Lycopodium when the urine has a deposit of pink urates.

Pulsatilla when the threshold to pain is low, and slight tension in the bladder provokes micturition.

Sarsaparilla when pain comes only at the end of micturition.

NOTES

NOTES

DANDRUFF

Also known as scurf, and officially as seborrhoea capitis.

Arsenicum Album very itchy scalp in persons with the typical Arsenicum personality (see Appendix).

Fluoric Acid dry scaling of the scalp, with marked loss of hair.

Graphites much scaling of the scalp, often with moistness and crusting, like impetigo.

Mezereum much itching, and with thick white crusts.

Oleander a minor remedy, but mentioned by Clarke as having a peculiar symptom – 'biting itching'.

Sepia moist dandruff.

Sulphur dandruff provoking much scratching, especially at night.

DEAFNESS

Some of the many forms of deafness, of many different causes, are not amenable to treatment. Some are benefited by surgery, and the persistent catarrhal forms of deafness are particularly suitable for homoeopathic treatment.

Borax for chronic suppurative otitis media, when antibiotics have not been completely successful.

Causticum with tinnitus and reverberation of the voice.

China Offic. for elderly debilitated persons with deafness and much tinnitus.

Kali Mur. for eustachian catarrhal obstruction.

Lycopodium with discharge from the ears, and eczema of the outer ear.

Mercurius has proved valuable in the treatment of 'glue ear'.

Nitric Acid when hearing is better in noisy surroundings.

Pulsatilla catarrhal deafness, better in the open air.

Silica catarrhal deafness with sinusitis as well.

DEBILITY

Every day hundreds of patients tell their doctors they have 'no energy' – usually an understandable exaggeration, really meaning that they have no zest – for many different reasons. Provided that debilitating diseases and psychological factors have been excluded, one of these homoeopathic remedies may restore the strength and enthusiasm required.

Arnica for those who feel battered and bruised.

Arsenicum Album weakness, faintness and loss of appetite.

Calc. Carb. 'cold and blue' – cannot get warm enough to get going; like a sluggish engine.

Calc. Phos. debility after acute illness.

Carbo Veg. debility after long and exhausting illness.

Kali Carb. weakness felt mostly in the back, probably signifying the inability to carry one or more burdens.

Kali Phos. 'nervous prostration' – especially in adolescents who are 'burning the candle at both ends' – when the smallest task seems too much to attempt.

Mag. Carb. tiredness felt mostly in the legs and feet.

Nux Vomica falls asleep in the early evening, is irritable and dyspeptic.

Sepia for the person who has lost interest in the family and finds housework exhausting, especially washing-up and laundry.

Silica when the diet seems adequate, but does not provide the energy one expects.

DELIRIUM

Aconite worse at night, with much fear.

Agaricus worse at night and with headache.

Arsenicum Album worse after midnight and very restless.

Baptisia disorientated and flushed.

Belladonna with high fever, dry red skin, and dilated pupils.

Bryonia with fever, vivid dreams and muttering.

Hyoscyamus foolish laughter alternating with muttering.

Lachesis worse at night, very talkative and with tight sensations in the neck and the chest.

Lycopodium worse from 4 p.m. to 8 p.m., with confusion over words.

Rhus Tox. with muscle pains and sudden episodes of weeping.

Stramonium muttering delirium and writhing movements.

Veratrum Album with much pain.

NOTES

NOTES

DELIRIUM TREMENS

This complication of alcoholism usually requires treatment in hospital, but it may be possible to give one of the following remedies as first aid:

Antim. Tart. for delirium with gastric pain and vomiting with much mucus.

Arsenicum Album very restless and agitated.

Belladonna furious delirium with staring eyes.

Hyoscyamus a quieter delirium, with muttering.

Nux Vomica with muscle spasms and twitchings.

Stramonium imagines he (or she) sees animals or insects.

DEPRESSION

This is a complicated subject, especially when one has to consider the extent to which anxiety and other emotions are mixed with depression. Sometimes the cause is obvious and can be dealt with simply; at other times psychiatric advice is necessary. In any case, the homoeopathic remedy can be administered as supplementary aid. Of the many which are valuable, only a few can be mentioned here:

Anacardium depression, with out-of-character swearing.

Arsenicum Album restless and self-reproaching.

Aurum Met. 'under a black cloud' and potentially suicidal.

Calc. Carb. for depression with fears of various kinds.

Ignatia full of contradictions.

Lilium Tig. worse in the evenings; tends to throw things about.

Lycopodium dyspeptic, melancholic and talkative.

Natrum Mur. weeps in solitude.

Nux Vomica for depression alternating with bad temper.

Pulsatilla can't fight against circumstances and doesn't care who sees her weeping.

Staphisagria easily upset by mere trifles and is resentful.

Sulphur depressed to the point of 'I don't care'.

DESPAIR

Aurum Met. for melancholia, when the patient wanders about saying little or nothing, and contemplates suicide.

Calc. Carb. for indecision, lack of confidence, despair of recovery – and undue sensitivity to cold.

Stannum when the patient has a sallow face, sunken eyes, is hypochondriacal, and loses hope relatively slowly.

DIARRHOEA

If this is not due to colitis, sprue or other diseases which need investigation and dietary advice, these are some of the remedies which may be helpful:

Arsenicum Album simultaneous diarrhoea and vomiting.

Bryonia due to sour fruit.

Colocynth with much colic, causing the patient to bend double.

Dulcamara after exposure to cold and damp.

Merc. Corr. slimy offensive stools with traces of blood, and with tenesmus.

Natrum Sul. morning diarrhoea, with stools of normal colour, but loose and urgent.

Petroleum worse after cabbage and other green vegetables.

Podophyllum watery yellow stools early in the morning, with a sense of weakness in the rectum.

Pulsatilla worse at night, and variable – no two stools alike.

Sulphur with much offensive flatus, smelling of bad eggs.

DISTENSION OF ABDOMEN

This is a symptom with many causes: some, such as baked beans, quite trivial; others, such as ascites, very serious. If investigations are needed, while waiting for the results, try one of these remedies:

Argentum Nit. with flatulence, and fondness of sugar.

Carbo Veg. wind accumulates in the stomach and is difficult to bring up.

China Offic. fullness in the abdomen, not better for belching.

Lycopodium dyspepsia similar to peptic ulceration, and a feeling of fullness even after only a little food.

Magnesium Phos. distension with colic, or colic with distension.

Millifolium distension due to ascites.

Pulsatilla frequent eructations, and nausea, and compulsion to loosen the clothing.

Raphanus 'incarcerated flatus' which will not move up or down in spite of much rumbling.

Sulphur distension due to flatus which is offensive.

NOTES

NOTES

DYSMENORRHOEA

Actea in stout and red-faced women.

Belladonna worse when lying down; the patient prefers to keep going.

Borax pain radiating down the thighs.

Caulophyllum with much cervical spasm in the first day or night.

Chamomilla angry – 'this is not fair' – 'I can't bear it'.

Cuprum Met. with cramps in the pelvis and in the fingers.

Lachesis worse on waking and worse after taking coffee.

Mag. Phos. with spasmodic pains and cramps, relieved by hot water bottles.

Pulsatilla with a flow of rather dark blood, and when the pain reduces the patient to tears.

Sepia with scanty flow and with dragging sensations in the pelvis.

Viburnum Op. when the periods are delayed and there is much pain, though there is little loss.

DYSPEPSIA

If indigestion is persistent, it is wise to consider investigation to exclude peptic ulcer and other serious conditions which may need surgery.

Argentum Nit. with eructations of wind and acid – eats too much sugar.

Calc. Carb. especially after fatty and oily food, very fond of boiled eggs, which upset.

Carbo Veg. acidity with much flatulence, in chilly persons who nevertheless like fresh air.

Dioscerea with colic, which is better for straightening or even leaning backwards.

Lycopodium with distension after only a little food, and developing pain which raises suspicion of a peptic ulcer.

Muriatic Acid when there is hyperacidity, especially if lots of antacids have been taken.

Nux Vomica easily upset by many things – alcohol, noise, arguments and so on. Pain occurs typically two hours after food.

Pulsatilla with nausea, leading to vomiting of watery material with mucus.

Robinia constant eructations and vomiting of intensely acid food residue, mostly at night.

Sulphur with regurgitation of food and acid, about one hour after meals; needs something at 11 a.m.

DYSPHAGIA

If painful or difficult swallowing is persistent, investigation will be needed to exclude organic lesions and neurological causes.

China Offic. with much sensitivity – the patient dislikes the throat being touched.

Gelsemium slow difficult swallowing, because the muscles feel weak.

Ignatia globus hystericus – says he or she cannot swallow – but does.

Kali Carb. slow swallowing, with choking.

Lachesis when there is a sense of constriction in the throat and neck (and chest).

Merc. Sol. with slimy mucus, hard to clear and swallow.

Nitric Acid with sharp sticking pains in the throat, as if due to a fish bone.

Phosphorus with burning pain, and traces of blood when the throat is cleared.

Stramonium with dryness of the throat and spasms of the muscles of swallowing.

EARACHE

In selecting the remedy, much depends on the nature of the ache or pain, and on the patient's reaction to it, as well as the cause of the trouble and the modalities. Some of the more important remedies are:

Apis when there is much swelling of the meatus.

Belladonna when throbbing is a feature.

Chamomilla for the child who reacts angrily.

Graphites when there is much smelly discharge.

Hepar Sul. when there is pus forming – before it is discharged.

Lachesis when swallowing markedly increases the pain.

Merc. Sol. worse at night.

Nitric Acid for sharp stabbing pains.

Nux Vomica when the patient is irritable and intolerant of noise.

Pulsatilla for earache caused by eustachian catarrh.

Sulphur when the meatus is red and itchy.

NOTES

NOTES

ECZEMA

The constitutional remedy is usually needed. Sometimes the causative agent in potency is valuable. In addition, one of the following remedies may be indicated:

Alumina dry irritating eczema.

Antim. Crud. eczema of the face and of the genitals.

Bovista eczema of the back of the hands.

Cicuta eczema of the chin.

Graphites eczema of the palms.

Hepar Sul. moist lesions, very sensitive to the touch.

Kali Sul. very similar to Pulsatilla – see the Appendix.

Mezereum eczema of the scalp, with much exudate.

Petroleum eczema which cracks easily, especially behind the ears.

Radium Brom. eczema after radiotherapy.

Rhus Tox. eczema with vesicles

Sulphur dry, itching and warm.

EXCITEMENT, AILMENTS AFTER

This section is mainly concerned with children who cannot settle down after parties and other exciting occasions – not illness, but a definite problem in some children.

Capsicum headache and disturbance of vision.

Coffea cannot get off to sleep.

Ignatia as a result of grief, alternate laughter and tears.

Kali Phos. mainly for adolescents who become overtired from excessive mental and physical exertion.

Nux Vomica stuttering.

Phosphoric Acid weakness, and trembling legs.

Pulsatilla easily excited to tears.

Staphisagria speechless with excitement, and then stammers.

FAINTING

Ordinary first aid measures are required for any faint; there is seldom time or need to give a homoeopathic remedy. But when faintness persists or recurs:

Aconite fainting due to fright.

Arnica after injury.

Arsenicum Album due to debility, with or without anaemia.

Carbo Veg. very cold and faint – has been called the 'corpse reviver'; at other times, gasping for air.

Cocculus as a result of travel sickness.

Hepar Sul. very sensitive to any pain.

Ignatia hysterical, and after over-breathing.

Iodum faint from hunger, when meals are delayed.

Nux Vomica faint at the sight of blood.

Pulsatilla fainting in hot stuffy rooms.

FEAR

Experience suggests that homoeopathic remedies for phobias are not mere placebos, but are effective when other measures such as tranquillisers have had little or no positive effect. These are some of the remedies which can be helpful:

Aconite fear of death; wakes suddenly in fright.

Argentum Nit. fear causing diarrhoea.

Gelsemium school phobia.

Kali Carb. fear of being alone, especially in the evening.

Opium 'petrified' – fear causing a state of helpless inaction.

Phosphorus fear of the dark, sensitivity to thunder storms, and nightmares.

Pulsatilla fears leading to floods of tears.

NOTES

NOTES

FEET, BURNING

Though this not a formal diagnosis, it is a tiresome symptom, not uncommon, and it is good to be able to offer something in addition to foot baths and foot powders:

Apis with swelling, and stinging sensations also.

Chamomilla hot and sweating feet.

Graphites burning sensations in the soles, worse when walking.

Medorrhinum also gets cramps and often sleeps in the knee-elbow position.

Phosphorus burning sensations, especially in the soles, and a tendency to haemorrhages elsewhere.

Pulsatilla hot sensations in the feet, extending up to the calves, and worse when the feet hang down.

Secale burning sensations in the hands as well as the feet.

Silica burning feet at night, and cold clammy feet by day.

Sulphur burning feet, worse at night – the patient often puts the feet out of bed to cool them.

FRIGHT, EFFECTS OF

Homoeopathic remedies can help as first aid after frightening episodes or situations. They can also help when the reaction persists for days or even weeks.

Aconite palpitations.

Belladonna nightmares.

Coffea insomnia.

Gelsemium diarrhoea or incontinence, or both.

Hyoscyamus delirium at night.

Ignatia hysterical behaviour, including convulsive movements.

Opium stupor and inaction – 'scared stiff'.

GALL BLADDER COLIC

This may need surgical treatment; while investigations are being arranged, one of the following will be helpful:

Berberis with obstruction, leading to putty-coloured stools and jaundice.

Calc. Carb. for the classical 'fat, fair and forty' women.

Chelidonium when the pain radiates in the typical manner to the right scapula.

China Offic. for pain leading to some degree of shock – with cold clammy skin, chills and rigors.

Colocynth pain relieved by flexing the back and legs, actually pressing on the painful area.

Dioscerea better when the back and legs are extended.

Lycopodium worse between 4 p.m. and 8 p.m.

Mag. Phos. pain in relatively short spasms, better for heat of hot water bottle.

GINGIVITIS AND PYORRHOEA

It is usually wise to obtain the advice of a dentist.

Arsenicum Album with a desire for frequent small drinks.

Borax when there are ulcers on the tongue and cheeks.

Calc. Phos. swollen, tender and easily bleeding gums.

Carbo Veg. sore bleeding gums and loose teeth.

Causticum toothache and ulceration of the gums.

Kali Carb. with offensive breath.

Merc. Sol. when the gums are swollen and not close to the teeth; bad breath.

Natrum Mur. if there is a bitter taste and loose teeth.

Nitric Acid when there are sharp pains like splinters and when ulceration develops.

Phosphorus for gums which are soft and 'spongy' and bleed easily.

Silica when gumboils develop slowly and heal slowly.

GLANDS, ENLARGED LYMPHATIC

The cause of the enlargement must be determined. In addition to any other necessary treatment:

Arum Triphyllum especially for submaxillary glands.

Barium Carb. associated with tonsillitis.

Calc. Carb. when the mediastinal glands are affected and cause cough and other symptoms.

Hepar Sul. for particularly tender glands, as in the axillae.

Merc. Sol. if suppuration threatens or occurs.

Silica when enlargement is slow and subsidence is also slow.

NOTES

NOTES

GLANDULAR FEVER

This infection is an example of the general principle that one does not treat a disease according to its label, but in consideration of its symptoms and signs. Those of glandular fever are: fever, malaise, sore throat, enlarged lymphatic glands, a rash which may look like measles or scarlet fever, tiny points of bleeding in the skin, and sometimes enlargement of the spleen and liver. The selection of the remedy is made according to whichever features of the illness are predominant at the time. Later on the constitutional remedy is usually needed, especially if convalescence is slow.

GOUT

Modern conventional treatment is usually necessary for the acute phases. The homoeopathic constitutional remedy is valuable in the intervals. Various other remedies are worth considering as an addition to control therapy:

Benzoic Acid when the urine is strongly coloured and smells rather like a stable.

Colchicum the classical remedy, usually the first to be tried when the constitutional remedy is not obvious.

Ledum better in cold air and better for cold bathing.

Lycopodium this is the constitutional remedy most often needed, especially if one foot is hot and the other is cold.

Pulsatilla when the pains go from one joint to another.

GRINDING OF TEETH

Of course this is not an illness, but it is a tiresome symptom or habit, and potentially harmful to the teeth.

Apis during fevers, especially if the uvula is swollen.

Belladonna during fever, with hot red dry skin.

Cicuta when associated with fits.

Cina when the child has threadworms, Cina can be given while waiting for the worms to be eliminated.

Podophyllum when there is intestinal colic as well.

Zincum Met. when the child is unduly fatigued.

HAEMORRHOIDS

Piles usually respond well to **Hamamelis** or **Paeonia** in ointment form. The ointments are equally soothing for internal as well as external piles. When they keep recurring, it is worth considering the use of remedies by mouth.

Aesculus with backache and prolapse of the rectum.

Aloe piles 'like grapes', associated with explosive diarrhoea.

Ammon. Carb. worse during the menses.

Capsicum with tenesmus and colic.

Causticum very tender piles.

Collinsonia also with tenesmus.

Hamamelis with soreness like a bruise.

Hypericum very sensitive, and bleeding easily.

Merc. Viv. with blood and mucus.

Nitric Acid with pricking sensations and with fissure.

Nux Vomica with irritability.

Paeonia much pain during and after bowel action, and often with a fissure.

Pulsatilla with mucus.

Ruta with prolapse of the rectum.

Thuja when the patient also has warts.

Verbascum with much irritation in the rectum.

HAIR, LOSS OF

Aurum Met. does not really care if all the hair falls out – is tired of life.

Fluoric Acid the hair goes dry and brittle and falls out.

Mercurius with constitutional disturbances – the patient is weak, tremulous and sweaty.

Mezereum the hair becomes curly and then falls out.

Selenium the pubic hair falls out as well as the scalp hair.

Sepia for the patient who is depressed and worried, especially about the family and by the family.

Thallium with a tendency to conjunctivitis.

NOTES

NOTES

HALITOSIS

If the breath remains tainted in spite of advice on oral hygiene and diet:

Aurum Met. 'putrid' breath, especially in girls at puberty.

Chelidonium when the liver is not working well and the tongue has a thick yellow coat.

Kreasote with gingivitis, when the gums are inflamed, spongy and bleed easily.

Nitric Acid with loose teeth, unhealthy gums and the weakness characteristic of all the acids.

Nux Vomica with sour-smelling breath, due to dyspepsia.

HANDS, DISORDERS OF

Actea rheumatic pains worse at night.

Apis acute swelling with much heat.

Argentum Nit. swelling of the hands, with numbness, especially at the menopause.

Bryonia swelling of the finger joints, without redness.

Calc. Carb. cold hands.

Caulophyllum pains in the wrists and fingers, with stiffness.

Fluoric Acid constantly moist palms.

Ledum boring pains in the thumbs, better when cool.

Rhus Tox. pains in most parts of the hands, especially in the thumbs of persons who do much knitting.

Ruta sprains of the wrists and fingers.

Sulphur hot hands.

HAY FEVER

The usual official name, allergic rhinitis, is not a full description because the eyes, the sinuses and the eustachian tubes are so often involved as well. The constitutional remedy is often needed. At other times it is helpful to prescribe the allergen in potency, or a nosode.

Allium Cepa much lachrymation.

Arsenicum Iod. dry sneezing and a wheezy chest.

Arundo much itching in the nostrils.

Dulcamara worse in the open air.

Euphrasia burning lachrymation.

Pulsatilla better in the open air.

Sabsdilla much itching in the nose, and chest symptoms, 'hay asthma'.

Sanguinaria hay fever complicated by polypi.

Silica nasal obstruction, worse on waking and with obstinate sinusitis – in chilly persons.

HEADACHE

No comprehensive list is attempted here; there are so many causes, and so many types. Nevertheless, it is worth presenting a short selection of some of the most useful homoeopathic remedies for headache.

Arnica after head injury, with or without concussion.

Belladonna 'bursting' headache, with dilated pupils.

Bryonia better for pressure and keeping still.

Gelsemium occipital headache and heavy eyelids.

Glonoine throbbing headache, sometimes due to too much exposure to the sun.

Lachesis worse on waking, and more on the left side.

Lycopodium with vertigo, and mainly on the right side.

Magnesium Phos. neuralgic pain, of a 'shooting, electric' type.

Nux Vomica the classical remedy for tension headache in the neck.

Pulsatilla better in the open air and after cold applications.

Sanguinaria headache gradually worse till noon, then improving.

Spigelia neuralgic pains, especially in the left temple.

Sulphur headache worse in the evening.

HEART DISORDERS

Heart failure should receive all necessary conventional treatment. Homoeopathic treatment is often a valuable supplementary measure. For symptoms which are tiresome and uncomfortable but not dangerous, the following remedies are worth remembering:

Apis relatively sudden pain in the heart with a sense of something like suffocation.

Arnica when there is a sensation that the heart is being squeezed.

Arsenicum Album palpitation and some irregularity, with much anxiety and restlessness.

Cactus the classical homoeopathic remedy for anginal pain, when the chest seems 'in a vice'.

Digitalis if the pulse is persistently slow, similar to the result of overdosage of digitalis glucosides.

Lachesis when pain in the heart extends to the neck.

Spigelia one of the most useful remedies, especially for strong palpitations, detectable by others and sometimes even reported to shake the bed.

NOTES

NOTES

HEARTBURN

A quaint word for one kind of dyspepsia, with burning sensations, for which the formal word is pyrosis.

Arsenicum Album if the symptoms are persistent, and associated with debility and loss of weight; investigation is needed.

Capsicum for burning sensations, not only in the stomach, but anywhere in the length of the bowel.

Cicuta when there is throbbing as well as burning.

Colchicum with nausea at the smell, sight or even thought of food.

Lycopodium burning pains with regurgitations or actual vomiting, as in peptic ulceration.

Phosphorus for the patient with burning sensations in the epigastrium and between the shoulder blades.

Sulphur when the symptoms are worse about 11 a.m., with belching as well as burning sensations.

HICCOUGH

Aethusa in infants who cannot tolerate much milk.

Arsenicum Album for hiccoughs associated with carcinoma of the stomach.

Cicuta in infants, especially if there have been convulsions.

Ignatia with other symptoms which are paradoxical and contradictory, raising suspicion of hysteria.

Ipecacuanha with much nausea.

Lycopodium with chronic dyspepsia and hyperacidity.

Mag. Phos. when the patient gets muscle spasms and neuralgic pains elsewhere, for instance cramps in the limbs.

Nux Vomica for hiccoughs occurring an hour or two after food.

Veratrum Viride if hiccoughs follows vomiting.

HYPERACUSIS

Unduly sensitive hearing is not a disease in the ordinary sense, but it is often mentioned as a secondary symptom, and can be useful in deciding the choice of the remedy:

Cannabis Ind. hearing very acute, combined with the exaggeration of duration of time and extent of space.

Coffea excessive sensitivity to music and voices, combined with active and alert thinking, and insomnia.

Nux Vomica the patient's own voice sounds unduly loud to him or her.

Opium undue sensitivity to sounds – an unexpected feature with the classical stupor.

Phosphorus small noises such as the screwing up of paper are 'intolerable', disturbing.

Silica loud noises actually cause pain in the ears.

Tabacum sensitivity to music and loud talking, with tinnitus as well.

HYPOCHONDRIASIS

Undue anxiety about one's health is sometimes an important factor in selecting the remedy.

Actea with depression, like a black cloud over everything.

Arsenicum Album anxiety drives him or her out of bed at night.

Aurum Met. thinks of suicide.

Calc. Carb. fears he or she will go crazy.

Ignatia with a tendency to hysteria.

Natrum Mur. melancholy, tired of life and wants to be alone.

Nux Vomica quarrelsome, and with episodes of violence.

Stannum with weakness, and symptoms predominantly abdominal.

Valerian when there are rapid irrational changes of mood.

HYSTERIA

Actea with gnawing sensations in the epigastrium.

Asafoetida with belchings and sensations of distension.

Crocus has emotional outbursts with quick repentance.

Ignatia with the classical lump in the throat.

Lachesis very talkative.

Moschus with difficult breathing and 'spasms' in the chest.

Platina haughtiness, with contempt.

Tarentula Hisp. with twitching or jerking of muscles.

Valerian excited and sleepless, sometimes with a sensation of floating in the air.

NOTES

NOTES

ICTHYOSIS

Dry scaly skin which has less than the normal amount of natural oil in it can predispose to infection, as well as being unsightly and uncomfortable. In combination with suitable creams to soften the skin, one of these remedies can be given by mouth.

Arsenicum Album dry skin with fine scales, thirsty for small drinks.

Graphites with cracks in the skin, usually overweight.

Natrum Mur. dry skin and an itchy patch on the nape of the neck.

Plumbum very little sweating and usually constipated.

Sepia with increased pigmentation.

Thuja for dirty looking skins, with warts.

IMPETIGO

This highly contagious skin disease, characterised by its purulent oozing which forms thick scabs, is usually treated by local antibiotic applications and should be covered to reduce contagion. Homoeopathic remedies are particularly helpful in resistant and recurrent cases.

Antim. Crud. for impetigo of the nostrils and the corners of the mouth.

Croton Tig. especially for impetigo of the scrotum.

Graphites when the oozing and the scabs are honey-coloured.

Hamamelis also for involvement of the scrotum.

Mezereum when the scalp is infected and thick crusts form.

Petroleum with cracks in the skin, especially behind the ears.

IMPOTENCE

Improving the general health by means of the best-indicated homoeopathic remedy may be a valuable factor in dealing with this trouble.

Agnus Castus ineffectual erection, with general debility and often with absent-mindedness.

Conium erections not sustained; and associated symptoms in the legs – cramps and coldness.

Graphites pains in the genitals, interrupting attempts at intercourse; unhealthy skin.

Lycopodium when it is anticipated that performance will fail; often with chronic dyspepsia.

Sepia for impotence associated with heaviness and dragging sensations in the genitals.

Sulphur if there is much itching and redness of the skin in the genital area, sometimes in association with alcoholism.

INFLUENZA

The nosode, **Influenzinum,** is valuable for prophylaxis. The constitutional remedy is valuable for delayed and slow convalescence. In the attack, the following remedies should be remembered:

Aconite in the first few hours of the illness.

Aesculus when the first symptom is backache.

Baptisia for delirium and confusion.

Bryonia when there is chest pain and pleural involvement, as in Bornholm disease.

Camphor when the stage of chill persists.

Eupatorium with pains in the bones.

Gelsemium with chills up and down the spine, and with heavy eyelids.

Glonoine with throbbing headache.

Pyrogen when secondary bacterial infection develops.

Rhus Tox. with muscle pains and stiffness.

Veratrum Album in very severe cases, with delirium, copious sweating, collapse and the rare 'heliotrope' cyanosis.

ITCHING

Agaricus with crawling sensations and sometimes associated with chilblains.

Calc. Carb. better for scratching.

Dolichos very itchy skin but with nothing abnormal to see.

Graphites when the patient scratches till the skin bleeds.

Manganum worse when sweating.

Merc. Sol worse on getting warm.

Mezereum much itching with development of scabs.

Psorinum scratching to the point of bleeding.

Rhus Tox. with urticarial lumps and bumps.

Rumex worse on undressing.

Sulphur worse on getting warm.

Urtica with urticaria, due to many substances in addition to nettles; for reactions to external irritants and to internal allergens.

NOTES

NOTES

JAUNDICE

A precise diagnosis is necessary – other treatment may be essential. In addition, one of these remedies may be helpful:

Chelidonium when there is also gall bladder pain, referred to the tip of the right scapula.

China Offic. for putty-coloured stools, flatulence and colic.

Crotalus may be helpful in haemolytic jaundice.

Hydrastis when the liver is palpably enlarged.

Mercurius with dull pains in the liver region and a nasty taste in the mouth.

Nux Vomica for dyspepsia, jaundice, itching skin and associated irritability.

Podophyllum if gall stones are present, causing obstruction and colic.

KNEES, PAIN IN

When fractures and other conditions which need surgical and other treatment have been excluded:

Apis for acute synovitis, worse for any form of heat.

Causticum when the knees cannot be fully extended, with tightness in the hamstrings.

Chamomilla better, surprisingly, when the joint is fully extended.

Kali Carb. for dull pains in the knees due to overweight, increasing the strain on the joints.

Ledum when caused by cold and damp; also after penetrating injuries by stings and by needles.

Natrum Mur. for prepatellar bursitis – 'housemaid's knee'.

Rhus Tox. for synovial effusions, with much protective stiffness of the surrounding muscles.

LARYNGITIS

Laryngitis which persists for more than a few days needs investigation. While waiting for the result or, more hopefully, to assist recovery:

Antim. Crud. for laryngitis due to heat.

Apis with oedema of the uvula and dysphagia as well.

Arnica after much shouting or other over-use of the voice.

Arum for laryngitis of singers, preachers and other public speakers.

Barium Carb. for simple chronic laryngitis.

Carbo Veg. for weakness of voice in old people.

Hepar Sul. in the later stages of bronchitis with laryngitis, when the cough has loosened but the hoarseness persists.

Lachesis for chronic laryngeal strain in very talkative people.

Phosphorus with irritating dryness of the throat and larynx, and sometimes specks of blood with the phlegm.

Rhus Tox. the voice improves with continued talking.

Spongia laryngitis with an associated dry 'barking' cough.

LEUCORRHOEA

If there is reason to suspect that there is infection which may have been acquired sexually, the disease is notifiable and should receive conventional treatment. In other cases, homoeopathic remedies should be considered, with special reference to constitutional features.

Alumina with raised itchy spots in the vagina.

Borax when the discharge is clear, like egg-white.

Carbo An. if the discharge burns the skin and stains the clothing yellow.

Kreasote yellow offensive discharge, causing itching and burning.

Medorrhinum for symptoms remaining after treatment of gonorrhoea.

Pulsatilla when the discharge is mucoid, rather like nasal mucus.

Sepia useful for prepubertal leucorrhoea, and also for cases in adults when there is much dragging sensation in the pelvic organs.

NOTES

NOTES

LIMBS: FIDGETY, JERKY OR RESTLESS

Fidgeting can be embarrassing; jerking, especially just when the patient is going to sleep, can be very annoying; and restlessness is often a valuable pointer to the similimum.

Fidgeting Kali Bich., Phosphorus or Zincum.

Jerking when going to sleep Agaricus, Belladonna, Ignatia, Kali Carb., Sepia.

Jerking as a result of sudden noise Borax, Carbo Veg., Opium.

General restlessness Arsenicum Album, Calc. Phos., Hyoscyamus, Pulsatilla, Stramonium, Tarentula.

LUMBAGO

Aconite as a result of exposure to draughts.

Arnica as a result of injury or when the muscles feel bruised.

Bellis Perennis worse after stooping in the open air, typically after gardening.

Berberis worse on waking.

Bryonia worse on any movement and markedly relieved by staying still.

Dulcamara worse after much stooping and exposure to cold and damp.

Nux Vomica after getting chilled.

Rhododendron worse when a storm is approaching.

Rhus Tox. when stiffness is a most marked feature and is gradually relieved by continued gentle motion.

MEASLES

This is a less serious problem nowadays, but cases still occur, and prompt treatment reduces the risk of complications.

Aconite in the early stages when frequent cough prevents sleep.

Belladonna for the child with very red face, headache, sore throat, before the sweating develops.

Bryonia when the rash is slow to appear.

Euphrasia if conjunctivitis is a prominent feature.

Kali Bich. when the cough produces stringy sputum and the voice is hoarse.

Mercurius when excess catarrh persists.

Pulsatilla for the child who is very sorry for himself or herself, with copious catarrh, and dislikes heavy bedclothes.

Sulphur if the rash is dusky and slow to clear.

The nosode, **Morbillinum**, is valuable for prophylaxis, and also for sequelae of measles, when the patient has never been really well since the infection.

MEMORY, IMPAIRED

It would be rash to claim that homoeopathic treatment would improve the memory, but the complaint of poor memory is a valuable clue to selecting the remedy for other disorders.

Aethusa poor memory and poor concentration.

Anacardium tends to swear because of the frustration caused by poor memory.

Barium Carb. absent-minded and inattentive.

Cocculus slow in remembering and easily distracted.

Lycopodium thinks his memory is worse than it really is.

Plumbum forgets words and is slow to grasp ideas.

Rhododendron thoughts disappear while they are being put into words.

Sulphur poor memory, especially for names.

MENOPAUSE, DISORDERS OF

Aurum Met. hot flushes and melancholia.

Glonoine throbbing in the head, with flushing.

Graphites flushing, especially of the face, sometimes with nose-bleeds and a tendency to put on weight.

Kali Carb. loss of appetite, regurgitations and backache.

Lachesis flushes, a sense of constriction round the neck, talkative; all symptoms worse on waking.

Sepia hot sweats, backache, especially in the sacral area, with sinking or dragging sensations.

Sulphuric Acid flushes worse in the evenings and after exertion; general weariness.

NOTES

NOTES

MENORRHAGIA

The cause of heavy periods should always be determined. While waiting for investigations:

Belladonna loss of bright red blood, in red-faced women.

Borax when the periods are early and profuse, with colic and nausea.

Bovista if the flow is worse at night.

Calc. Carb. for women who are pale, overweight and chilly.

Chamomilla with clots, and intolerance of pain.

China Offic. when the clots are dark.

Ferrum Met. better when walking about slowly.

Ipecacuanha bright loss, with nausea.

Phosphorus no clots and restless, fidgety.

Sabina intermittent loss.

Secale thin watery loss, with no clots.

Sepia with bearing down pains and a tendency to prolapse.

MENTAL EXHAUSTION (BRAIN FAG)

Aethusa distracted and exhausted by too much mental work of different kinds in rapid succession – confused.

Anacardium loss of memory or fear of loss, especially before exams.

Calc. Phos. after much worry or illness.

Gelsemium during or after influenza.

Kali Phos. in adolescence.

Lycopodium with confusion in choosing the right words.

Phosphoric Acid with physical weakness as well.

Picric Acid with indifference, little will power and persistent headache.

Silica with impaired memory due to overwork and with headaches, usually in the sinuses.

Zinc Met. with poor memory, after insufficient sleep, trembling and fidgeting.

MOUTH ULCERS AND VESICLES

Borax mouth ulcers with grey bases, very sore.

Hepar Sul. very sensitive vesicles, proceeding to ulceration with yellow base; gingivitis too.

Merc. Corr. ulcers, excess saliva and a bad taste.

Natrum Mur. Blisters like pearls.

MUMPS

In addition to the usual management and nursing required for the acute phase, homoeopathic remedies are helpful. The nosode, **Parotidinum**, is valuable when convalescence is slow.

Aconite in the early febrile stage.

Calc. Carb. for pale fat children.

Chamomilla when there is bad temper and intolerance.

Jaborandi this contains various alkaloids, including Pilocarpine, and is almost specific for mumps.

Phytolacca if there are neck symptoms and sore throat as well as the swelling of the parotid glands.

Pulsatilla if the testes become involved and orchitis develops.

MUSCLE PAINS

Aconite for stiff neck, especially if due to a draught of air.

Arnica for bruised muscles.

Bryonia for pain in the intercostal muscles, with or without involvement of the pleura.

Causticum for pain in the hamstrings, with limited extension.

Dulcamara for aching muscles due to cold damp conditions.

Ledum for muscles involved in stab wounds and hypodermic injections.

Nux Vomica for pain in the muscles at the back of the neck, associated with tension headaches.

Phytolacca for muscle pains in heavily built persons; especially for pain in the deltoids.

Rhus Tox. for painful stiff muscles.

NAILS, DISORDERS OF

Alumina for brittle and spotted nails.

Antim. Crud. for horny thick nails, especially toenails.

Arsenicum Album when the nails crack easily.

Calc. Carb. for soft nails which break off easily.

Graphites when the nails grow thick and distorted.

Secale when the nails separate easily from their beds.

Silica for brittle and yellow nails.

Thuja when the nails are brittle and when the patient also has condylomata or warts.

NOTES

NOTES

NAUSEA

A common symptom with many causes, and for which there are many homoeopathic remedies. The cause should be established before treatment is begun. These are some of the remedies most often used:

Arsenicum Album worse after midnight.

Calc. Carb. worse after drinking milk and in the morning.

Cocculus especially for travel nausea and sickness.

Colchicum very sensitive to the smell of cooking.

Ipecacuanha for persistent nausea, with headache as well.

Iris one of the remedies for migraine, when nausea is a pronounced feature.

Kali Carb. as a result of excitement and of motion.

Lobelia when there is much salivation with the nausea.

Nux Vomica worse in the morning, as with a 'hangover'.

Pulsatilla for nausea during pregnancy, better in the open air, often accompanied by much catarrh.

Tabacum better in the open air, away from tobacco smoke.

NECK, STIFFNESS OF

Aconite for acute torticollis due to draughts of cold air.

Calc. Carb. with hoarseness and enlarged neck glands.

Cicuta when the neck is stiff and turned to one side.

Dulcamara stiffness after a chill, better for hot applications.

Mag. Phos. sudden stiffness with neuralgic pains.

Nux Vomica for tension in the back of the neck, with tension headache and irritability.

Phytolacca stiffness due to sore throat, tonsillitis, quinsy, in muscular persons with 'bull neck'.

Rhus Tox. when the stiffness extends to the trapezius.

NEURALGIA

Aconite for facial neuralgia caused by cold draughts.

Arsenicum Album for intermittent burning neuralgic pains.

Chelidonium for intercostal neuralgia, worse from touch as well as worse from motion.

Colocynth for trigeminal neuralgia, especially if the pain has a 'tearing' quality.

Kalmia for neuralgia in the right side of the face and in the right arm.

Mag. Phos. for paroxysmal pains like electric shocks in the limbs, especially in the sciatic plexus.

Ranunculus Bulb. for intercostal and supraorbital neuralgias.

Spigelia for sudden sharp pains in the left temple, often with associated palpitations.

NOSE, DISEASES OF

This section is mainly concerned with bleeding from the nose. See also the sections on Catarrh and Sinusitis.

Arnica for bruising and bleeding after injury.

Belladonna red face, throbbing headache and bleeding.

Calc. Carb. when there are polypi with associated catarrh and obstruction.

Carbo Veg. for old people who sneeze a lot and then get nose-bleeds.

Ferrum Phos. especially for children whose noses bleed during feverish illnesses.

Hamamelis when nose-bleeds are frequent, and when there is engorgement of veins elsewhere, as in the legs.

Phosphorus frequent and profuse sudden nose-bleeds.

Pulsatilla polypi causing nasal obstruction.

Sanguinaria polypi, much sneezing and headaches.

Sulphur itching nose, causing much sneezing.

NOTES

NOTES

NUMBNESS

If numbness persists, a neurological assessment is needed.

Aconite numbness and tingling of the hands and feet as in the hyperventilation syndrome.

Chamomilla numbness of the hands, worse when grasping.

Conium numbness of the legs, beginning in the feet and working upwards.

Ignatia numbness of the heels, worse when walking.

Natrum Mur, numbness, tingling and exhaustion.

Phosphorus burnings and tinglings as well as numbness.

Secale numbness, coldness and threat of gangrene.

OBESITY

The essential treatment of obesity is, of course, advice on diet, habits and exercise. Obesity or the tendency to it is a valuable clue for finding the constitutional remedy for other disorders.

Calc. Carb. with enlarged glands.

Capsicum 'lax, lazy, fat and red' – with burning sensations anywhere in the alimentary system.

Ferrum red-faced and subject to dyspepsia.

Graphites with a tendency to skin diseases.

Hepar Sul. hypersensitive and liable to develop recurrent small boils.

Kali Carb. with backache and catarrhal tendencies.

OVARIES, DISORDERS OF

Actea ovarian pains at puberty.

Apis ovarian tenderness, especially on the left.

Colocynth ovarian neuralgia, associated with intestinal colic.

Hepar Sul. tenderness of the ovaries, part of a general hypersensitivity.

Lachesis pain mainly on the left, worse for tight clothing.

Lilium Tig. right ovarian pain, extending to the thighs.

PANIC

Aconite at night, on waking after bad dreams, during fever.

Argentum Nit. stage fright and exam 'funk'.

Arsenicum Album when alone.

Gelsemium shaking with fright.

Opium 'paralysed' by fright, unable to act.

Stramonium excessive fear of the dark.

PERSPIRATION AND BODY ODOUR

Arsenicum Album sweaty palms, worse in company.

Calc. Carb. sweating, especially of the head, in infancy.

China Offic. sweating and debility after illness.

Fluoric Acid the sweat has a sour smell.

Merc. Sol. when the sweat has an offensive odour.

Phosphorus exhausting sweats, especially at night.

Psorinum persistent bad odour in spite of washing.

Sepia excessive sweating, especially menopausal.

Silica cold sweaty feet.

Sulphur hot sweaty feet.

PHARYNGITIS

Apis with swelling of the uvula – can hardly swallow.

Belladonna when the pharynx is hot, dry and red.

Capsicum if there is a hot smarting sensation, as if caused by pepper.

Kali Bich. with the sensation of a hair stuck in the throat.

Lac Caninum when the soreness goes from one side to the other.

Lachesis if there is a bluish tinge of the pharynx, a sense of constriction, and dysphagia.

Merc. Cyan. when there is a grey exudate.

Merc. Sol. with much saliva and retching.

Nitric Acid if there are pricking sensations, as from a fish bone.

Phytolacca when there is a feeling of a hot lump in the throat, and swallowing causes pain which radiates to the ears.

NOTES

NOTES

PHLEBITIS

The risk of fragments of thrombus breaking off and causing embolism should always be remembered and guarded against. In addition to such measures, one of these remedies may be helpful:

Apis in the early stages, with pain, redness and swelling.

Arnica when the phlebitis is the result of known injury.

Fluoric Acid if there are hard 'knots' in the affected veins.

Hamamelis when the pain and tenderness is sufficient to cause lameness.

Hepar Sul. for marked sensitivity – when the patient can hardly bear any touching of the area.

Lachesis when there is a purple tinge of the affected area.

Vipera if there is a bursting sensation in the limb and if it is much worse when allowed to hang down.

PLEURAL PAIN

This title is chosen so as to include pain with or without fever or effusion – a broader collection of disorders – not just pleurisy in the usual sense.

Belladonna in the early stages of acute febrile pleurisy.

Bryonia the remedy most often needed for sharp pleural pains, better when lying still on the painful side.

Chelidonium when there is much coughing, with pain behind the sternum, referred from the mediastinum.

Hepar Sul. useful in later stages, when recovery is slow, and the chest is sensitive to cold air.

Natrum Sul. for pleural pain accompanied by dry cough, worse at night, better sitting up and pressing on the painful area.

Rumex when the pain is accompanied by tickling and raw sensation in the trachea.

Sticta for the patient who starts coughing and finds it very difficult to stop.

POLYPI, NASAL

Cadmium Sul. with a sense of tightness at the root of the nose.

Calc. Carb. with loss of sense of smell, and sometimes with swelling of the upper lip.

Phosphorus the polypi bleed easily when the nose is blown.

Psorinum with chronic post-nasal drip, especially in patients who tend to be chilly.

Pulsatilla with plentiful catarrh.

Thuja the remedy most often indicated for warts and other kinds of lumps on the skin, as well as for nasal polypi.

PREMENSTRUAL TENSION

Calc. Carb. tenderness of the breasts.

Causticum pessimistic and irritable.

Conium with sore breasts and cold legs.

Graphites distinct increase in weight.

Kreasote restless and irritable.

Lachesis when there is fluid retention and heaviness of the breasts.

Lycopodium cross and melancholic.

Natrum Mur. also for fluid retention; irritable and sad.

Nux Vomica very irritable and quarrelsome.

Pulsatilla weepy and with painful breasts.

Sepia depressed, irritable and with reduced libido.

PROSTATE, ENLARGEMENT OF

Eventually, surgery may be needed, but homoeopathic remedies may delay or even avoid the need for surgery.

Barium Carb. especially for thin under-weight persons, with frequency and a slow stream.

Calc. Carb. for heavy, sluggish and apprehensive men, when the prostate produces much mucus.

Conium when frequency is especially troublesome at night and worse after any alcohol.

Iodum if the gland is hard – and arouses suspicion of carcinoma, needing investigation.

Pulsatilla with itching and oozing of mucus from the meatus.

Sabal when there are stinging pains on micturition, and the bladder and urethra seem unduly irritable.

PRURITUS VULVAE

This tiresome, distressing and sometimes embarrassing complaint may be due to infection, and then will need appropriate conventional treatment. If there is no discharge:

Ambra itching worse at night.

Merc. Sol. much burning after scratching, and worse when wetted by urine.

Nitric Acid with pricking like needles, worse while walking.

Petroleum with visible dermatitis of the vulva.

Platinum with voluptuous crawling sensations.

Rhus Tox. when there are small vesicles and these are sometimes the manifestation of herpes.

 Sepia in slim brunettes, especially during pregnancy.

NOTES

NOTES

PSORIASIS

This is a constitutional disturbance of the skin, and needs a careful assessment of the whole person. The family history as well as the personal history are important.

Arsenicum Album see the Appendix on Constitutional Remedies.

Cicuta Vir. thick crusts with much burning and itching.

Clematis when pustules form in or under the scaly patches.

Graphites with thick gummy exudate indicating infection.

Kali Ars. if the itching is worse in the warm, and especially if there is more scaling than usual.

Petroleum when there is a history of use of ointments with a paraffin base.

Psorinum when the skin never seems really clean.

Sulphur see the Appendix.

RHEUMATISM

This section concerns the muscles, not the joints.

Arnica worse after bruising and over-exertion.

Bryonia worse for movement, better for rest and pressure.

Causticum better in damp weather; when there is a tendency to contracture, especially of the hamstrings.

Colchicum worse at night and in winter.

Dulcamara when caused by or aggravated by cold and damp.

Kali Iod. when the muscle pains are tearing or darting.

Ledum for muscle pains after stings, puncture wounds and injections.

Merc. Sol. worse at night and often with 'sour' sweat.

Pulsatilla for muscle pains which shift from place to place.

Rhus Tox. with much stiffness, especially of the hands and fingers; worse on starting to move, but soon better on continued movement.

Ruta for pains in tendons as well as in muscles.

SACRAL AND SACRO-ILIAC PAIN

Appropriate movements, exercises and manipulations are usually effective.

Aesculus sacro-iliac pain, worse when walking slowly or standing.

Agaricus with sensations of bruising, pressure or weight.

Aloe sacral pains accompanying diarrhoea and piles.

Berberis pain referred from the rectum.

Rhus Tox. when the pain results in marked stiffness – almost immobility.

Sepia with dragging sensations in the pelvis.

Sulphur when the pain extends to the groins.

Tellurium for pains shooting up from the sacrum and down to the thighs.

SALIVATION

Excess or deficiency of saliva is obviously not a disease, but can be a useful clue in helping to find the right remedy for other disorders.

Excess

Allium after eating – paradoxical.

Ipecacuanha with nausea and gagging as a result of coughing.

Iris with migraine or similar headache.

Merc. Sol. with sore gums – worse at night.

Nitric Acid with mouth ulcers and prickings.

Veratrum Album with cold sweat and faintness.

Deficiency

Arsenicum Album when the mouth is dry with fear.

Barium Carb. with numbness as well as dryness.

Belladonna when the mouth is hot and dry.

Bryonia little saliva, but little thirst.

Capsicum with burning sensations and dryness.

Carbo Veg. when the tongue is rough as well as dry.

Hyoscyamus in low muttering delirium.

Natrum Sul. if the tongue looks and feels slimy but dry.

Nux Moschata when there is so little saliva that the tongue sticks to the palate.

Silica if the mouth and tongue are dry in spite of a fair amount of thin saliva.

NOTES

NOTES

SCIATICA

Ammon. Mur. worse when sitting and the hamstrings feel short.

Arsenicum Album especially for older people.

Colocynth worse because of cold and damp.

Dioscerea better when the spine is extended.

Gelsemium worse when resting at night.

Kali Carb. when sciatic pain is made worse by coughing, especially about 3 a.m.

Lycopodium worse in the afternoon and when lying on the affected side.

Mag. Phos. for the classical 'electric' shooting pains down the leg, worse on coughing and better for flexion of the spine.

SCREAMING AND CRYING CHILDREN

First it is necessary to determine if there is any physical cause for screaming which requires treatment. These remedies are useful when there is a habit of apparently unnecessary screaming.

Antim. Tart. for crying, whining and frequent waking.

Belladonna during fever and delirium, and as a result of nightmares.

Calc. Carb. for the child who cries in his or her sleep.

Chamomilla cries angrily till picked up.

Cicuta when screaming leads to howling, then moaning, then weeping.

Cina for noisy delirium and dislike of even being looked at.

Phosphorus when nightmares cause screaming, especially in dark haired children.

Pulsatilla more for pitiful weeping, especially in fair haired children.

SHIVERING, CHILLS AND RIGORS

Aconite with fever.

Arsenicum Album with waves of icy coldness.

Astacus with urticaria due to shell fish.

Bellis Perennis as a result of having a cold drink when over-heated.

Camphor for the patient who asks alternately for warmth and then for cold air.

Carbo Veg. despite the shivering, wants the window opened so that he or she can sit in a draught.

Cinchona when fever and sweating is preceded by rigors.

SINUSITIS

Persistent or recurrent sinusitis, not responding well to other treatments, is often improved by the well-indicated homoeopathic remedy.

Agaricus when sinusitis causes widespread headaches.

Belladonna when there is pain, especially in the frontal sinuses, worse on stooping.

Graphites if blowing the nose leaves fairly prolonged pain.

Hepar Sul. when the catarrh is yellow and the face is hypersensitive.

Kali Bich. when the catarrh is stringy.

Kali Carb. when the catarrh is lumpy.

Pulsatilla when nasal obstruction is variable and causes pain above the eyes.

Silica when the pain feels as if it is in the bones surrounding the sinuses

Spigelia for sinusitis with neuralgic type of pain.

SKIN, CRACKS AND FISSURES IN

Alumina for the hard dry skin of old people, easily cracked – especially the hands.

Calc. Carb. when the skin cracks in the winter.

Graphites for cracks in the nostrils, on the lips, behind the ears, and of the nipples.

Nitric Acid when cracks bleed easily, and for cracks with crusts forming on the edges of the nostrils.

Natrum Mur. especially for cracks in the centre of the lower lip.

Petroleum for cracks in the skin of the palms and behind the ears, worse in winter.

Sarsaparilla for cracks in the skin of the feet, and of the hands, fingers and thumbs, and at the corners of the mouth.

Sepia 'the washerwoman's remedy' – for cracks resulting from prolonged immersion in water.

Sulphur for intertrigo – cracks or splits in the skin folds, when the skin is softened, macerated, and often infected.

NOTES

NOTES

SLEEP, DISTURBANCES OF

Aconite very restless sleep, twisting and turning and undoing the bedclothes.

Arnica unable to sleep because overtired, and the bed feels hard.

Belladonna when the limbs jerk just as the patient is getting off to sleep; also for nightmares.

Calc. Carb. for the child who cries or moans in sleep; also when there is marked sweating of the head during sleep.

Coffea kept awake by continuing thoughts: 'Can't switch off'.

Ignatia yawns a lot but can't get off to sleep.

Kali Carb. wakes about 3 a.m. and can't get back to sleep.

Nux Vomica insomnia because of dyspepsia, eventually sleeps, but wakes with a 'hangover' or something very like it.

Opium deep sleep lasting longer than normal, hard to rouse.

Phosphorus when there are frequent nightmares.

Sambucus wakes gasping for breath, as if suffocating.

Spigelia kept awake by palpitations, which are sometimes strong enough to disturb the partner.

Sulphur needs an extra pillow to reduce a sense of congestion in the head; the limbs get unpleasantly hot, and the patient sticks them out of bed.

SMELL; SENSE OF SMELL DIMINISHED

It would be rash to claim that homoeopathic remedies can alone restore the full sense of smell, but when catarrh is obviously a factor in the problem, they are likely to be helpful.

Anacardium when there is nasal obstruction.

Calc. Carb. when polyps are present.

Hepar Sul. when there is yellow catarrh, a tendency to sweating and an improvement in warm weather.

Influenzinum as a consequence of influenza.

Phosphorus with burning sensations and a tendency to nosebleeds.

Pulsatilla when the amount of catarrh varies markedly from hour to hour, and is better in the open air.

Sepia with dryness of the nasal passages.

Silica when there is associated sinusitis.

SPRAINS

Arnica for sprains involving the wrist or ankle, especially when there is a haematoma.

Calc. Phos. for sprains of the carpus.

Rhus Tox. for sprains in rheumatic subjects, with much stiffness and reluctance to move.

Ruta for most sprains – almost a specific.

STAMMERING

The essential treatment of stammering and stuttering is speech therapy, to encourage good breathing and good phonation. But homoeopathic remedies can be helpful as well.

Belladonna especially for children who talk too fast.

Causticum when stammering is accompanied by grimacing.

Merc. Sol. with tremors, especially of the tongue.

Nux Vomica for the patient who is 'jumpy' and irritable, and tends to omit or transpose syllables as well as stammering.

Stramonium when there are exaggerated movements of the limbs while talking.

STIFFNESS OF MUSCLES AND OF JOINTS

Apis for stiffness due to synovitis.

Arnica for stiffness after exertion and strenuous games.

Bryonia stiffness of elbows and knees, better when quite still.

Calc. Sul. when the stiffness is in the shoulders.

Causticum stiffness around the knees and ankles, with tightness of the hamstrings, preventing full extension of the knees.

Chelidonium when the legs are stiff, heavy and lame.

Ledum for stiffness due to cold and damp.

Rhus Tox. for stiffness which is worse on first movement, improving during continued movement, especially in the wrists, hands, fingers and thumbs.

Silica for stiffness associated with scars.

NOTES

NOTES

STROKES

The old name apoplexy is best avoided. The relatively new term, CVA, cerebral vascular accident, is not really appropriate because a stroke is not an accident, but a lesion. Hospitals are often reluctant to admit patients with strokes until they have survived the first forty-eight hours. Meanwhile, homoeopathy can help.

Arnica often chosen because the cerebral lesion is similar to a bruise, a haematoma.

Belladonna when the face is flushed and there is throbbing headache.

Natrum Mur. when the face is pale and there is throbbing headache.

Nux Vomica when the stroke occurs after a heavy meal or too much alcoholic drink.

Opium when the patient is unconscious, breathing heavily, and the face is dusky or cyanosed.

Sulphur for the heavy red-faced beer-drinking type.

Veratrum Album when the clinical picture is one of 'collapse' – shocked, sweating and cold.

STYES

Graphites when the styes produce much sticky honey-coloured exudate, as occurs with impetigo.

Phosphorus when there is twitching of the eyelids, and a burning sensation in them.

Pulsatilla when the eyelids are stuck together on waking.

Staphisagria when there is frontal headache.

Staphylococcinum when infection with staphylococci is proved, or suspected, and styes persist, this nosode can be expected to stimulate the development of better resistance to the germs.

Thuja Hahnemann's chief antipsoric remedy.

SUNSTROKE

This is a convenient term to include the ill-effects of over-exposure to the sun, and also the ill-effects of other forms of heat.

Aconite with fever, confusion and apparent stupidity.

Antim. Crud. after too much exertion in the sun.

Belladonna with throbbing headache, hot dry skin and dilated pupils.

Cuprum Met. when much sweating has caused excess salt loss and cramps.

Gelsemium with giddiness, as if intoxicated.

Glonoine with throbbing headache, flushed face and sweating.

Natrum Mur. when the patient is irritable and hates any fuss.

SYNOVITIS

Effusion into a joint often causes some instability. This applies especially to the knee, and it is usually wise to support the knee with a crêpe type of bandage.

Apis in the early stages, when the joint is painful, hot and swollen.

Arnica when there is evidence or suspicion of bleeding into the joint.

Belladonna when the pain is eased by hot applications.

Bryonia especially for synovitis of small joints.

Causticum for subacute or chronic synovitis, with associated weakness of the joint.

Colchicum for acute synovitis, especially of the legs, with hot tearing pains, like gout.

Pulsatilla for hot swellings, especially of the elbow and of the knee, with the swelling visible above the patella.

Rhus Tox. for effusion and stiffness of the surrounding muscles.

Ruta for traumatic synovitis associated with sprains.

TEETHING TROUBLES

Actea when nervous and restless during teething.

Borax for teething complicated by aphthous or ulcerative stomatitis; and when there is dislike of downward motion, when being put into the cot.

Calc. Carb. when teething is late, and associated with diarrhoea and green stools.

Calc. Phos. for babies who are late in teething, late in sitting up and late in walking.

Chamomilla fretful and angry – yells till picked up and is quiet until put back in the cot.

Kreasote when the teeth have poor enamel which begins to decay soon after eruption.

Merc. Sol. when there is excess salivation during teething, sore gums and diarrhoea.

NOTES

NOTES

TEMPERAMENT AND MOOD

The constitutional temperament and the mood of the moment can be useful guides to the correct remedy for psychological disturbances and for many disorders with a predominantly somatic manifestation. Homoeopathic remedies are often valuable alternatives to conventional tranquillisers, anti-depressives and anxiolytics.

This list shows only one remedy for each temperament or mood, leaving room for the reader to make additions as required.

Angry Chamomilla.

Apathetic Phosphoric Acid.

Company wanted Phosphorus.

Company shunned Natrum Mur.

Complacent Arnica.

Confused Baptisia.

Despairing Aurum.

Excitable Belladonna.

Frightened Aconite.

Haughty Platinum.

Humble Pulsatilla.

Hurried Lilium Tig.

Hysterical Ignatia.

Impatient Sulphur.

Indifferent Sepia.

Irritable Nux Vomica.

Lamenting Lycopodium.

Lazy Calc. Carb.

Obstinate Tub. Bov.

Quarrelsome Petroleum.

Raging Hyoscyamus.

Resentful Staphisagria.

Restless Arsenicum Album.

Sad Stannum.

Taciturn Silica.

Talkative Lachesis.

TESTES, DISORDERS OF

Arnica after injury and bruising.

Aurum Met. chronic neuralgic pain, causing depression.

Belladonna acute 'intolerable' pain.

Clematis persistent chronic pains extending to the groins and the thighs.

Hamamelis when the testes are very sensitive, and when the skin of the scrotum is disordered.

Pulsatilla acute pain with much swelling, as in mumps.

Rhododendron aching in the testes, worse before thunderstorms.

Spongia persistent aching due to much coughing.

THIRST, ABNORMAL

When diabetes (mellitus or insipidus) have been excluded, consider:

Arsenicum Album wants to drink little and often.

Belladonna when the mouth is hot, dry and red.

Bryonia for thirst for large quantities.

Dulcamara wants hot drinks, but they are vomited.

Phosphorus thirsty for cold drinks, which are soon vomited.

Stramonium wants sour drinks such as lemon juice.

Sulphur is thirsty but not hungry.

THRUSH (APHTHOUS STOMATITIS)

Antim. Tart. for children, especially when they vomit milk.

Arsenicum Album marasmic cases, with ulcers and prostration and low fever, especially if there is simultaneous vomiting and diarrhoea.

Borax for simple stomatitis, with established ulcers – the old-fashioned Borax in Glycerine was unwitting, or unacknowledged, homoeopathy.

Capsicum with hot sensations in the mouth, made worse by cold water.

Kali Chlor. with salivation and tenderness of the salivary glands.

Merc. Sol. with salivation and slimy diarrhoea.

Natrum Mur. with herpetic vesicles on the lips.

TINNITUS

Noises in the head or in the ears of a purely subjective origin are usually resistant to treatment, and it is rash to hold out hopes of a cure. Sometimes the well-chosen remedy can bring some relief:

China Offic. for tinnitus associated with deafness, and sometimes with headache and vertigo.

Graphites for tinnitus associated with the so-called 'boiler-maker's deafness' – when the hearing is better in a noise.

Lachesis when the noises are most pronounced on waking.

Petroleum for noises of a whizzing nature, as of a breeze.

Phosphoric Acid for tinnitus associated with debility, weakness and vertigo.

Pulsatilla when the noises are worse when there is upper respiratory catarrh.

Spigelia for tinnitus with neuralgic pains in the ears, intermittent rather than continuous.

 Sulphur when the noises are worse at night.

NOTES

NOTES

TONGUE, DISORDERS OF

The tongue is abnormal in many diseases – in some anaemias and as a result of various infections. The possibility of malignant changes must be remembered.

Aconite tingling or numb.

Antim. Crud. lumpy and tender – in old people who do not feel the cold.

Apis swollen and redder than usual – often associated with oedema of the uvula.

Arsenicum Album with a sore red tip.

Arum cracked and bleeding.

Belladonna dry and reddened.

Bryonia dry and pale, even nearly white.

Cantharis scalded or burned.

Hydrastis burned, raw and with prominent taste buds.

Merc. Sol. swollen, slimy or moist, and indented by the teeth.

Natrum Mur. patterned – sometimes called 'geographical'.

Rhus Tox. with a sore red tip – especially if there is pain, stiffness and cracking in the jaw joints.

TONSILLITIS

Acute attacks of tonsillitis may need antibiotics. Chronic or recurrent tonsillitis usually responds well to homoeopathy.

Barium Carb. for undersized children with recurrent attacks.

Calc. Carb. for fat chilly children with a tendency to persistent enlargement of the cervical glands.

Hepar Sul. with much inflammation and yellow exudate, when the soreness is better for warm drinks.

Lachesis with marked dislike of anything touching the throat, causing a sense of constriction.

Lycopodium also with a sense of constriction and when the symptoms are worse about 4 p.m. to 8 p.m.

Merc. Sol. when there is marked sweating, bad breath and extra salivation.

Nitric Acid with much exudate and with pricking sensations.

Phytolacca when the neck is swollen and tender as well as the tonsils – the so-called 'bull neck'.

Sulphur when the tonsils remain large in between attacks, almost touching in the midline; for children who are noticeably 'warm blooded', in contrast to those who need Calc. Carb.

TOOTHACHE

Apis with swelling of the gums.

Bryonia when the teeth feel too long.

Calc. Carb. pain worse for cold air or cold drinks.

Calc. Fluor. when the dental enamel is deficient.

Chamomilla worse when in bed.

Coffea better for cold water.

Kali Carb. worse when eating.

Mag. Phos. neuralgic pains like little electric shocks.

Plantago when the teeth are sensitive to touch and cold air.

Pulsatilla worse for warm drinks, better in the open air.

Staphisagria when the teeth are blackened and crumbling.

Obviously, any homoeopathic first aid should be followed by a visit to the dentist.

TRACHEITIS

Apis with a sensation of swelling in the trachea.

Arsenicum Album dry, burning and irritating, as if constricted.

Bryonia worse for talking, smoking and in warm rooms.

Calc. Carb dry tracheitis, worse in the evening and when speaking.

Cannabis Sativa worse in the morning, with sticky mucus.

Capsicum crawling and tickling in the trachea causing sneezing as well as coughing.

Carbo Veg. worse in the evening.

Causticum tearing sensations on coughing.

Kali Bich. irritation in the nose, larynx and trachea, with stringy mucus.

Lachesis worse after sleep and when touched.

Nux Vomica tickling, worse when exhaling.

Phosphorus cough, hawking and rawness, worse in the evening and after cold drinks.

Rumex soreness worse in cold air.

Silica mucus coughed up, especially soon after meals.

Stannum sweetish yellow mucus coughed up.

Sulphur constant irritation, worse at night.

NOTES

NOTES

TRAVEL SICKNESS

This can sometimes be incapacitating, and even dangerous; homoeopathic remedies can control and cure it without causing the drowsiness which is often a side effect of conventional treatment.

Aconite with restlessness and fear of accident or disaster.

Apomorphine when vomiting occurs with little or no warning.

Borax for nausea which is worse during downward movement, as in aircraft, and also in lifts.

Cocculus almost a specific for travel sickness, especially when there is vertigo and a sense of emptiness in the head.

Petroleum when nausea is accompanied with eructations of wind from the stomach.

Tabacum with cold sweat and prostration.

TREMORS

Actea tremors of the legs, making walking difficult.

Agaricus rhythmic spasms of groups of muscles, especially of the neck.

Antim. Tart. tremors of the limbs with coldness of the hands and feet.

Gelsemium tremors of the whole body, with hot and cold shivers up and down the spine.

Ignatia tremors combined with gross jerking movements.

Merc. Sol. tremors of the fingers and of the tongue, with stammering.

Stramonium tremors persisting after a fright, with writhing movements as well.

ULCERS

This section refers to ulcers of the skin only.

Arsenicum Album with burning pains, better for warmth.

Belladonna when the surrounding skin is very red and hot.

Hamamelis for ulcers associated with varicose veins.

Kali Bich. when ulcers have a 'punched out' look, with clear-cut edges.

Lachesis for ulcers with a purple tinge around them.

Merc. Sol. when there is much oozing of pus and serum.

Mezereum when scabs form too readily and pus collects under the scabs.

Nitric Acid for ulcers which bleed easily, and when there are sharp pains like splinters.

Phosphorus for ulcers which bleed easily.

Silica when ulcers are slow to develop and slow to heal.

URETHRAL SYNDROME

This section concerns pain on passing urine in the absence of any infection in the bladder, and felt most in the urethra.

Arsenicum Album burning pain causing agitation – unable to keep still because of the pain.

Camphor most pain at the beginning of micturition, due to tenesmus at the neck of the bladder.

Clematis when the urine passes slowly and intermittently, in men more often than in women.

Phosphorus when urine is passed in small quantities and sometimes with specks of blood.

Sepia for women more often than for men, and especially for pain due to caruncle.

Silica when there is urethral stricture.

Terebinth especially for children when spasms of pain occur just before the urine begins to pass.

URINATION, DISORDERS OF

Apis burning stinging pain while passing urine, which is scanty and concentrated.

Berberis when there is mucus in the urine, either as a floating film or as a sediment.

Cantharis scalding pain and frequency.

Causticum for frequency in old people, day and night.

Conium intermittent flow.

Kali Carb. slow starting, due to prostatic enlargement – helpful while waiting if operation is necessary.

Lilium Tig. frequent urging and with dragging sensations.

Nux Vomica for the irritable bladder, in irritable people, resulting in frequency which may be exaggerated.

Petroselinum sudden urging – any delay causes agony.

NOTES

NOTES

URINE, INCONTINENCE OF

This problem occurs mostly in childhood, but also at other ages.

Apis incontinence with stinging and burning, sometimes as a result of coughing.

Arsenicum Album during pregnancy.

Belladonna at night, especially if the urine becomes very concentrated.

Causticum in old people, who hardly feel the urine passing.

Equisetum in childhood, at night.

Fluoric Acid mainly in the daytime.

Merc. Corr. seems to pass more than is drunk – often associated with tenesmus.

Natrum Mur. takes more salt than most people.

Phosphoric Acid as a result of coughing – more in the day than at night.

Pulsatilla during pregnancy, often while walking.

Sulphur with burning sensations in the urethra.

URINE, RETENTION OF

Homoeopathic remedies are helpful as first aid, but a surgical opinion will be needed if the trouble persists or recurs.

Apis when there is oedema of the penis obstructing the urethra.

Arnica for retention of urine after injury.

Causticum for retention after surgical operation for any abdominal trouble.

Natrum Mur. for the patient who cannot pass urine in the presence of anyone.

Nux Vomica when there is an urge to pass urine every few minutes, but no success.

Opium retention of urine with no pain and no desire to empty the bladder.

Tarentula when the patient cannot sit still and relax and allow the urine to flow.

URTICARIA

Acute cases are best treated with **Apis** if the lesions are mainly on the face, or by **Urtica** if the lesions are on the limbs.

Apis burning and stinging, especially with oedema of the eyelids and the lips.

Croton when there is more itching than burning, especially of the genitals, male or female.

Dulcamara for urticaria involving mainly the lower half of the body.

Lycopodium for chronic or persistent urticaria, worse between 4 p.m. and 8 p.m.

Natrum Mur. when the lesions develop after strenuous exercise.

Nux Vomica with mental irritability and intolerance, leading to much scratching.

Rhus Tox. burning and itching, sometimes with vesicles.

Rumex worse when undressing.

Ruta when there is dyspepsia as well as urticaria.

Sulphuric Acid if accompanied by the typical soreness of acid burns.

Urtica for true nettle rash, but also valuable as first aid for urticaria due to other plants.

UTERINE PROLAPSE

This condition usually needs surgical treatment or some form of support. Homoeopathy is often helpful.

Arctium Lappa for prolapse with much bearing-down sensation.

Argentum Nit. when there is ulceration, which needs other treatment as well.

Calc. Carb. when noticably worse after lifting things.

Lilium Tig. 'hurried and worried' – the typical mother and housewife.

Kali Carb. with much backache, especially since the birth of a baby.

Palladium better during social occasions and worse after.

Platinum for prolapse with associated cramps and spasms, especially in haughty superior persons.

Pulsatilla when prolapse is felt more during menstruation.

Sepia the remedy most often indicated for prolapse, with dragging sensations, worse after washing clothes or bathing children, and consequent depression.

NOTES

NOTES

VARICOSE VEINS

In addition to support stockings, adequate rest and elevation, and other measures, think of these remedies:

Arnica when the veins have been bruised or feel bruised.

Calc. Carb. when the patient is over-weight, chilly, subject to cramps in the calves and feet.

Carbo Veg. when the peripheral circulation is sluggish, even to the extent of cyanosis.

Fluoric Acid one of the principal remedies for varicose veins, especially if they are tender and 'knotty'.

Hamamelis for varicose veins associated with haemorrhoids.

Pulsatilla particularly useful during pregnancy, when some degree of pelvic pressure impedes the venous circulation.

VERTIGO

This section refers to true vertigo with a rotatory sensation, not to mere faintness.

Belladonna worse when turning in bed.

Borax with fear of downward movement.

Bryonia with vomiting – better keeping still.

Calc. Carb. worse when looking up.

China Offic. with tinnitus and debility.

Cocculus for vertigo associated with travel sickness.

Conium worse when lying down.

Gelsemium with trembling.

Kali Carb. better in the open air.

Natrum Mur. with headache.

Nux Vomica with nausea.

Pulsatilla with catarrh.

VOMITING

This is a symptom of many different causes, and if it persists an accurate diagnosis must be made. As first aid and while waiting for investigations:

Aethusa when babies or children cannot digest milk without vomiting – different from mere regurgitation.

Antim. Tart. with much rattling bronchial catarrh which is swallowed and then vomited.

Arsenicum Album for simultaneous vomiting and diarrhoea.

Cuprum Met. when vomiting is accompanied by spasms and cramps in the abdominal muscles.

Ipecacuanha when nausea persists after vomiting, especially during pregnancy.

Iris for watery vomiting accompanying migraine.

Nux Vomica if vomiting occurs two or three hours after meals.

Pulsatilla after rich and fatty foods.

Sulphur with hot sensations in the chest – retrosternal.

Another helpful approach to the problem of selecting the remedy can be based on the following sections:

Due to **Anger** Chamomilla, Colocynth, Nux Vomica.

Due to **Cough** Aluminium, Antim. Tart., Bryonia, Drosera, Hepar Sul., Ipecacuanha, Kali Carb.

With or alternating with **Diarrhoea** Argentum Nit., Arsenicum Album, Veratrum Album.

After any **Drink** Antim. Crud., Arsenicum Album, Bryonia, Phosphorus, Tabacum, Veratrum Album.

After only a little **Food** China Offic., Ipecacuanha, Phosphorus, Sepia, Silica, Sulphur.

With **Headache** Ipecacuanha, Melilotus, Pulsatilla, Sanguinaria.

During **Pregnancy** Asarum, Chelidonium, Ignatia, Kreasote, Lactic Acid, Natrum Sul.

Due to **Travelling** Bryonia, Cocculus Indicus, Petroleum, Tabacum.

NOTES

NOTES

WARTS (VERRUCAS)

Calc. Carb. multiple warts, horny and itchy.

Causticum multiple warts, especially on the face and on the eyelids.

Dulcamara large smooth fleshy warts.

Kali Mur. warts on the hands.

Natrum Carb. warts which become macerated and ulcerated.

Natrum Mur. warts on the palms.

Nitric Acid 'cauliflower' warts which itch, prick and bleed easily.

Sepia large hard pigmented warts.

Sulphur hard painful warts.

Thuja the most useful remedy for warts in general, almost a specific.

WHITLOW

Infections around the finger nails can lead to some deformity if they are neglected. In addition to the usual nursing procedures and surgical measures, and antibiotics if necessary, one of the following remedies will be valuable treatment:

Belladonna when the finger is very hot and throbbing.

Fluoric Acid if there is a sensation as of a splinter under the nail.

Hepar Sul. with much throbbing, worse at night and better for holding the hand up.

Lachesis if there is a blue or purple tinge surrounding the infection.

Silica when the infection is relatively slow in developing.

WHOOPING COUGH

Antim. Tart. when there is much catarrh, causing 'rattling' sounds in the chest.

Arnica when the child cries out because of the pain of coughing.

Coccus. Cacti when the sputum is stringy, hanging from the mouth in lengths.

Cuprum Met. when there are cramps and even convulsions, as happens sometimes in babies.

Drosera when the cough is worse after midnight.

Hepar Sul. when the paroxysms of coughing are brought on by draughts.

Ipecacuanha when gagging and vomiting follows the coughing.

Kali Carb. when the patient is left exhausted by the cough.

Spongia when the cough sounds rather like a dog barking.

In addition, the nosode, **Pertussin**, is valuable as prophylaxis and also for sequelae, if convalescence is slow.

WOUNDS AND OTHER INJURIES

Arnica for bruises.

Calendula for abrasions and grazes, to encourage the regrowth of the epithelium.

Cantharis for burns and scalds.

Hepar Sul. for wounds and injuries which develop infection.

Hypericum for crush injuries involving damage to nerves, especially of the fingers and toes.

Ledum for puncture wounds – insect stings, needle pricks and stab wounds by wood, metal or other substances.

Rhus Tox. for muscle injuries causing much stiffness.

Staphisagria for pain persisting in surgical wounds.

Symphytum for encouraging union of fractures.

NOTES

NOTES

APPENDIX - OUTLINE DESCRIPTIONS OF THE MOST IMPORTANT CONSTITUTIONAL REMEDIES

Dr Marion Gray, BM, BCh, MRCGP, MFHom

This Appendix is provided to enable the reader to identify certain salient characteristics of a patient's total personality, or 'constitution'. This comprises a combination of the physical type, the psychological features, and the reactions to the environment and events.

The personality patterns and the diseases to which they are prone are described under the name of the remedies. It is commonplace in homoeopathy for a patient to be described by the constitutional remedy which most closely suits his or her personality (e.g. a 'Sulphur type', or a 'Sepia type').

Each remedy on the following pages is described in a standard form for ease of reference. First there is a general description of the personality, then a few of the more important modalities (factors which make the condition better or worse). This is followed by typical likes and dislikes of food and drink. Finally, there is a list of the clinical diagnoses indicating the main range of action, provided the complete personality picture conforms.

In general, the constitutional remedies should be used for chronic or recurring diseases. It may happen, for example, that Belladonna is successfully prescribed for a single case of acute otitis media. However, if the child suffers from several episodes of this infection, a constitutional remedy should be sought to prevent further trouble.

It should be stressed that only the most basic information has been provided here to suggest the most likely remedy. It may well be necessary to confirm the choice by reference to a detailed textbook of homoeopathic materia medica.

ARSENICUM ALBUM

(Arsenic trioxide)

These patients are usually anxious, pale, thin individuals. They are very sensitive and fastidious. They are also intelligent and quick in mind and body. If ill, their prostration is out of proportion to their condition, and often accompanied by irritability. Their pains are burning in nature.

Chilly

Right-sided

Modalities
Better for heat.
Worse soon after midnight.

Food
Wants frequent small drinks.
Likes fat.

Conditions in which indicated
Acute colds – fluent watery discharge from the nose causing a sore upper lip.
Diarrhoea and vomiting – especially if occurring at the same time.
Asthma.
Acute heart failure – especially at the early stage.

CALC. CARB.

(Natural calcium carbonate from the middle layer of oyster shells)

These patients are flabby persons who sweat easily on the head and chest. They tend to get depressed easily, and are slow both mentally and physically. They worry a great deal and are forgetful. They even fear that they might lose their reason.

Chilly

Modalities
Dislikes open air.
Worse for cold.

Food
Dislikes milk.
Enjoys eggs.

Conditions in which indicated
Enlarged glands.
Faulty bone development – delayed dentition, exostoses and spurs, rickets.
Depression.
Constipation – feels better when constipated. Unlike the similar remedy Graphites, which feels worse when constipated.
Gallstones.
Rheumatism – often follows Rhus Tox. well.

NOTES

NOTES

CAUSTICUM

(Potassium hydrate)

The Causticum patient is a broken down, despondent, anxious person who dislikes mental exertion.

Chilly

Right-sided

Modalities

Better for damp, warm weather.
Worse for cold, dry winds.

Food

Worse for sweet foods.
Worse for coffee.

Conditions in which indicated

Paralysis of single nerves, e.g. Bell's palsy, Horner's syndrome.
Hoarseness – worse in the morning.
Conditions affecting the jaw and mouth. Pain may be referred to the ear.
Rheumatism – contractures of tendons; stiff necks, especially those brought on by draughts.
Urinary difficulties – stress incontinence, frequency.
Warts – on face and finger tips.

GRAPHITES

(Carbon, black lead)

These people are coarse-featured with a tendency to obesity. Their skin is rough, dry and may be cracked. They are indecisive, timid and startle easily. Depression is a common state of mind. Constipation is frequently found. They sometimes complain of an odd sensation as if they felt a cobweb on their face. They are fat, chilly and have a tendency to constipation.

Chilly

Modalities

Better in the dark.

Food

Worse for seafood and fish.
Worse for meat.
Worse for sweet foods.

Conditions in which indicated

Skin – eczema or rashes with sticky secretions like honey, often behind the ear or at the margins of mucous membranes. There may also be crusting.
Digestion – stomach pains relieved by eating. Digestive symptoms and skin complaints may strangely alternate.
Glands – enlarged.
Nose-bleeds – following flushes.

HEPAR SUL.

(Calcium sulphide. Interior of oyster shells burnt with flowers of sulphur)

These are irritable, touchy, over-sensitive people. They sweat easily, but do not like to uncover themselves, preferring to pull a blanket around themselves.

Chilly

Modalities
Better for warm wet weather.
Worse for touch.
Worse for uncovering.
Worse for cold air.

Food
Likes sour food, pickles and condiments.

Conditions in which indicated
Suppuration – profuse secretions smelling like old cheese, e.g. abscesses, infected ulcers, etc.
Tonsillitis – rapid enlargement of glands; sensation of plug or splinter in the throat; pain may be referred to the ear.
Cough and croup.

IGNATIA

(St Ignatius bean)

The emotional aspects of this remedy are of fundamental importance. These patients are nervous and neurotic. Their mental and physical conditions change rapidly and they often present with what seems a contradictory symptom picture.

Chilly

Modalities
Better for heat.
Worse for grief.
Worse for worry.

Food
Desires sour, acid foods.

Conditions in which indicated
Effects of grief.
Hysteria.
Throat – sensation of a lump in the throat. This is better for swallowing, especially solids.
Headaches – worse for coffee; as if a nail had been driven through the side of the head.

NOTES

NOTES

KALI BICH.

(Bichromate of potash)

This remedy is well suited to the fat, chubby, sluggish patients who present with ropey, stringy discharges. Pain is characteristically felt in circumscribed small areas. Alternatively, the pains may migrate and alternate with other symptoms (e.g. stomach pain may alternate with catarrh).

Chilly

Modalities
Better for heat.
Worse around 2 a.m.–3 a.m.
Worse for beer.
Worse for undressing.

Food
Craves beer.
Likes starch and potatoes, but these upset.

Conditions in which indicated
Chronic catarrh – with tough stringy discharges and crust formation.
Stomach pain – fullness immediately after eating; worse for beer; may be associated with a punched-out ulcer, e.g. a peptic ulcer.
Rheumatism – pains that wander from one place to another.

KALI CARB.

(Potassium carbonate)

This remedy is well-suited to the patient who is full of fears. It also has an element of irritability and great weakness associated with it. The patient may well express a feeling of failure in life, together with distressing forgetfulness. Physically the Kali Carb. type is flabby and sallow, sometimes with flat feet. The impression is one of weakness and depression.

Chilly **Right-sided**

Modalities
Better for motion.
Worse for touch and easily startled. Worse at 3 a.m. Worse after coition. Worse lying on the left, and on the painful side.

Food
Likes sweet and starchy foods. Likes acid and sour drinks.

Conditions in which indicated
Lungs – asthma. Cough and pneumonia – pain is independent of respiration, often right sided, worse for pressure, better for leaning forward, dry cough with little sputum.
Headache – bitemporal.
Backache – after pregnancy; before menses.
Digestive – flatulence and distension; worse for ice-cold water.

KALI PHOS.

(Potassium phosphate)

This remedy is especially good for the nerves of thin, dark haired, exhausted neurotics. (All Kali salts are fat except Kali Phos.) These patients hate to be alone and yet are very shy and find they are worse for talking to people. They often feel as if they are going to break down.

Chilly

Modalities
Better for motion.
Better for heat.
Worse for food.
Worse for worry.
Worse for exertion.
Worse for excitement.

Food
Craves ice-cold water.
Likes sweet foods.
Likes sour foods.

Conditions in which indicated
Headaches – typically in overworking students; the head is tender to the touch.
Insomnia – in adolescents.

LACHESIS

(Venom of the Surukuku snake)

The person requiring Lachesis is usually very loquacious and excitable. There is often a lot of jealousy and suspicion associated with this remedy. An interesting feature is the inability to tolerate tight clothes around the neck. Another marked feature is the blue or purple colour of any skin disorder.

Warm **Left-sided**

Modalities
Better for the onset of discharges, e.g. nosebleeds, menstruation. Worse after sleep. Worse for pressure (except headaches).

Food
Craves alcohol. Likes oysters. Likes coffee.

Conditions in which indicated
Sore throats – left-sided; purplish tinge to the throat – often looks less bad than the pain would suggest; worse when swallowing, especially hot fluids; empty swallowing may be more painful than swallowing solids; pain may be referred to the ear.
Hot flushes.
Headaches – hammering; from the effects of the sun (follows glonoine well); better for pressure.
Retinal haemorrhages in diabetes.

NOTES

NOTES

LYCOPODIUM

(Club moss)

These people are usually of a reserved and intellectual disposition, but lack physical stamina. They may be tall and thin, and often have a worried expression on their face which results in a furrowed brow. They are sensitive and conscientious people who, although disliking company, dread total solitude. They are subject to anticipatory fears, and get worried about impending responsibilities and public performances, etc.

Chilly
But dislikes 'stuffy' warmth.

Right-sided

Modalities
Worse 4 p.m.–8 p.m.
Worse for tight clothing.
Worse for over-eating.
Hungry, but easily satiated.

Food
Likes sweet foods.
Likes warm drinks.

Conditions in which indicated

Digestive and liver disorders – flatulence; chronic ulcers.

Respiratory tract – neglected or slowly resolving right-sided pneumonia; post-influenzal debility.

Urine – may have a pink sediment.

Sore throat – right sided (may subsequently go to the left); better for warm drinks and worse for cold drinks.

MERCURIUS

(Black oxide of mercury)

This remedy is characterised by the offensiveness of all discharges, and is useful for people 'filthy in both mind and body'. They are sweaty (the sweat is oily and may stain the bedclothes), weak and tremulous. The tongue is flabby and shows the imprint of the teeth. There may also be spongy, bleeding gums. Much saliva is produced and there is a metallic taste in the mouth.

Modalities
Worse for sweat.
Worse for the warmth of the bed.
Worse at night.

Food
Thirsty for cold drinks.

Conditions in which indicated

Sore throats – with visible exudate on the tonsils. (In the past it was used for diphtheria.)

Glands – enlarged; mumps.

Diarrhoea – green slime; blood; tenesmus during and after evacuation.

Skin – ulcers; itching and stinging.

NATRUM MUR.

(Common salt)

These patients often have sallow, greasy, spotty complexions, with fine, oily hair. They tend to depression and are unstable and touchy. They hate fuss, but dislike to be ignored.

Chilly

Modalities
Worse at 10 a.m.
Worse by the sea.
Worse in the sun.

Food
Thirsty.
Desires salt.

Conditions in which indicated
Depression.
Headache – hammering; migraines.
After shock and grief.
Skin – acne; herpes; urticaria; eczema, especially around the hair margin on the head.
Palpitations.
Irregular menstruation.

NUX VOMICA

(Poison nut which contains strychnine)

This is the remedy for the irritable patient, who is quarrelsome, hates contradiction and is inclined to get angry. He is hypersensitive to noise, light and smell. He is often an epicurean and connoisseur of wine, and typically leads a sedentary life.

Chilly

Modalities
Better for warmth. Better for being alone. Better in the rain.
Worse in the dry, windy weather. Worse two hours after eating. Worse in the open air. Worse for the sun.

Food
Likes piquant food. Likes fat.

Conditions in which indicated
Gastro-intestinal tract – hiatus hernia; indigestion from overindulgence; diverticulitis; constipation – frequent ineffectual desire to defaecate; rectal problems, e.g. haemorrhoids.
Onset of common cold – esp. if it starts with a scratchy throat.
Headache – on waking, e.g. 'hangover'; worse after sun.
Backache – acute lumbago – has to sit up to turn over in bed.
Hiccough.

NOTES

NOTES

PHOSPHORUS

The Phosphorus individual is intelligent, bright and sensitive. Physically, he is often tall and slender. He is imaginative, and this may lead to certain fears, e.g. the dark, of being alone, thunder, etc.

Chilly **Right upper and left lower complaints**

Modalities
Better for eating – may have night hunger. Better for warmth, except the head and stomach. Better for rubbing.

Food
Desire for salt and spices. Thirsty for cold drinks – these may be vomited when they become warm in the stomach.

Conditions in which indicated
Haemorrhage – bright red blood, e.g. epistaxis.
Respiratory tract – cough (hard dry); asthma; pneumonia – often right lower lobe, worse lying on unaffected side.
Vomiting – can be useful for vomiting of pregnancy.
Headache – migraines, but appetite is not impaired.

PULSATILLA
(Wind flower)

This remedy is suited to sandy haired individuals, with a tendency to gaining weight easily. They are shy, gentle people (commonly women) prone to tearfulness and changeable moods.

Chilly
Some authorities say warm. Certainly they are averse to heat.

Modalities
Better in the fresh air.
Better for gentle motion.
Better for sympathy.
Worse for a stuffy atmosphere.

Food
Rich foods and fat disagree.
Thirstless.

Conditions in which indicated
Catarrh – thick bland yellow or green discharge.
Menstrual problems – menses late at puberty; dysmenorrhoea.
Styes.
Varicose veins.
Skin – eczema; urticaria.
Difficulty controlling micturition, e.g. enuresis.
Arthritis.

SEPIA

(Ink of the cuttlefish)

This remedy is well suited to the depressed, indifferent, worn-out person (usually a woman). The Sepia patient is averse to sympathy and company, yet dreads to be alone. Physically, she is often dark haired and has a rather sallow skin.

Chilly

Modalities
Better for food. Better for sleep. Better for exercise, especially dancing. Enjoys a thunderstorm. Worse for tobacco smoke.

Food
Nausea at the thought of food. Dislikes milk, especially if boiled. Loathes fat. Desires vinegar and sour foods.

Conditions in which indicated
Gynaecological – dragging down sensation in the pelvis, better for sitting with crossed legs; menstrual disturbances; menopausal symptoms, e.g. flushes.
Depression – often associated with the menstrual cycle or menopausal problems.
Headache – migraine; headache over the left eye.
Skin – brown patches; ringworm; herpes; urticaria; falling hair, often with an itchy scaly scalp.

SILICEA

(Flint)

This is well suited to the pale-faced, thin, delicate 'china-doll' type person, with small sweaty hands and feet. The Silicea patient appears gentle and even 'spineless' but can be peculiarly obstinate at times. They panic easily at the thought of responsibility, due largely to their feeling of inadequacy and their dread of failure.

Chilly

Modalities
Better for warmth.
Better for wrapping up (often tight).
Worse for thought of pins and sharp objects.
Worse for draughts.

Food
Poor appetite.
Prefers cold food.
Dislikes meat.
Thirsty.

Conditions in which indicated
Boils.
Expulsion of foreign bodies, e.g. splinters.
Disorders of the bones, teeth and nails.
Respiratory tract – chest infections that do not clear up; recurrent problems that originate from pleurisy years back.
Headache – occipital – may travel forwards often to settle over the right eye; better for warmth and being tightly wrapped; may follow mental stress.
Constipation – the 'bashful stool' which is difficult to expel.

NOTES

NOTES

SULPHUR

The Sulphur patient may either be a lank, lean, dyspeptic person with a predisposition to meditation and philosophy, or an active well-fed lover of life. Whatever the type, cleanliness is not a strong point and he will commonly look dishevelled. He is also selfish and has no regard for others.

Warm
Burnings, especially on the soles of the feet.

Modalities
Better for the open air.
Worse for a bath.
Worse for the heat of the bed.
Worse 11 a.m. – sinking feeling.
Worse for standing.

Food
Always hungry.
Likes fat.
Likes sweet foods.
Thirsty.

Conditions in which indicated
Skin – eczema; boils.
Burning pains.
Diarrhoea – that drives the person out of bed in the morning.
Haemorrhoids.
Catarrh.

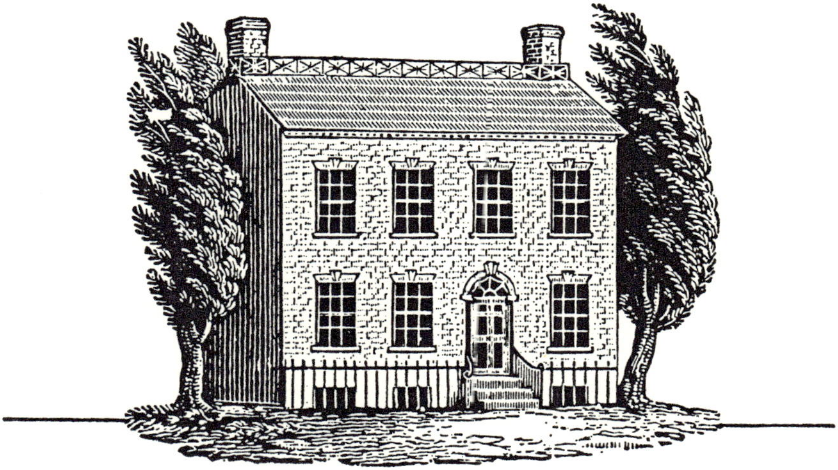

THE TRUE HEALING ART

List of Pharmacies and Companies in the United States and Canada that Can Supply Homeopathic Remedies

(Courtesy of the National Center for Homeopathy,
Falls Church, Virginia 22042)

CALIFORNIA

City Pharmacy
1435 State Street
Santa Barbara, CA 93101

College Pharmacy
90 N. Ashwood Avenue
Ventura, CA 93003

Horton and Converse
621 West Pico Boulevard
Los Angeles, CA 90015

Mylans Homeopathic Pharmacy
222 O'Farrell Street
San Francisco, CA 94102

Nutri-Dyn
717 S. Bristol Ave.
Los Angeles, CA 90049

Santa Monica Drug
1513 Fourth Street
Santa Monica, CA 90401

Standard Homeopathic Company
436 West 8th Avenue
Los Angeles, CA 90014

Village Drug Store
Ojai, CA 93023

ILLINOIS

Ehrhart and Karl
17 N. Wabash Ave.
Chicago, IL 60602

MARYLAND

Washington Homeopathic Pharmacy
4914 Delray Avenue
Bethesda, MD 20014

MISSOURI

Luyties Pharmacal Company
4200 Laclede Avenue
St. Louis, MO 63108

NEW JERSEY

Humphreys Pharmacal Company
63 Meadow Road
Rutherford, NJ 07070

NEW YORK

Keihl Pharmacy, Inc.
109 Third Avenue
New York, NY 10003

Weleda, Inc.
841 South Main Street
Spring Valley, NY 10977

PENNSYLVANIA

Boericke and Tafel, Inc.
1011 Arch Street
Philadelphia, PA 19107

John A. Borneman and Sons
1208 Amosland Road
Norwood, PA 19074

VIRGINIA

Annandale Apothecary
7023 Little River Turnpike
Annandale, VA 22003

CANADA

D. L. Thompson Homeopathic Supplies
844 Yonge Street
Toronto 5, Ontario
Canada M4W 2H1